Math Basics for the Health Care Professional

Math Basics for the Health Care Professional

Third Edition

Michele Benjamin Lesmeister, MA

Renton Technical College
Renton, Washington

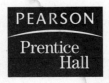

PEARSON

Prentice
Hall

Upper Saddle River, New Jersey 07458

Library of Congress Cataloging-in-Publication Data

Benjamin Lesmeister, Michele.
    Math basics for the health care professional / Michele Benjamin
Lesmeister. — 3rd ed.
            p. ; cm.
    Rev. ed. of: Math basics for the healthcare professional / Michele
Benjamin Lesmeister. 2nd ed. 2005.
    Includes bibliographical references and index.
    ISBN 978-0-13-512632-5 (alk. paper)
    1. Medicine—Mathematics.   2. Mathematics.   3. Medical sciences.   I. Math basics
for the healthcare professional.   II. Title.
    [DNLM: 1. Mathematics.   2. Allied Health Personnel—education.   3. Drug
Dosage Calculations.   QT 35 B468m 2008]

R853.M3B46 2008
510—dc22   2007048554

Notice: Care has been taken to confirm the accuracy of information presented in this book. The authors, editors, and the publisher, however, cannot accept any responsibility for errors or omissions or for consequences from application of the information in this book and make no warranty, express or implied, with respect to its contents.

    The authors and publisher have exerted every effort to ensure that drug selections and dosages set forth in this text are in accord with current recommendations and practice at time of publication. However, in view of ongoing research, changes in government regulations, and the constant flow of information relating to drug therapy and drug reactions, the reader is urged to check the package inserts of all drugs for any change in indications of dosage and for added warnings and precautions. This is particularly important when the recommended agent is a new and/or infrequently employed drug.

Publisher: Julie Levin Alexander
Publisher's Assistant: Regina Bruno
Executive Editor: Mark Cohen
Associate Editor: Melissa Kerian
Editorial Assistant: Nicole Ragonese
Managing Production Editor: Patrick Walsh
Production Liaison: Cathy O'Connell
Production Editor: Vikas Kanchan, TexTech
Manufacturing Manager: Ilene Sanford
Manufacturing Buyer: Pat Brown
Senior Art Director: Maria Guglielmo
Art Director: Chris Weigand
Cover Designer: Kevin Kall
Director of Marketing: Karen Allman

Marketing Manager: Harper Coles
Marketing Specialist: Michael Sirinides
Media Development Editor: John J. Jordan
New Media Project Manager: Stephen Hartner
Image Resource Center Director: Melinda Patelli
Rights and Permissions Manager: Zina Arabia
Visual Research Manager: Beth Brenzel
**Cover Visual Research & Permissions
    Manager:** Karen Sanatar
Image Permission Coordinator: Ang'john Ferreri
Composition: TexTech International
Printer/Binder: Bind-Rite Graphics
Cover Printer: Phoenix Color Corp./Hagerstown
Cover Image: Medioimages/Photodisc

Pearson Education, Ltd., *London*
Pearson Education Australia Pty. Limited, *Sydney*
Pearson Education Singapore Pte. Ltd.
Pearson Education North Asia Ltd., *Hong Kong*
Pearson Education Canada, Ltd., *Toronto*

Pearson Educación de Mexico, S.A. de C.V.
Pearson Education—Japan, *Tokyo*
Pearson Education Malaysia, Pte. Ltd.
Pearson Education, Upper Saddle River,
    New Jersey

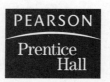

10 9 8 7 6 5 4 3
ISBN-10: 0-13-512632-0
ISBN-13: 978-0-13-512632-5

For Max and Thresa Benjamin—the masters of encouragement, perseverance, and inspiration.

Contents

Preface for Educators and Learners

Math Basics for the Health Care Professional was written to serve a large population of learners preparing for careers within health occupations as well as those working toward employment upgrades in the field. Suggested specific applications of this work text are high school vocational programs; adult education programs that prepare students for health fields; self-study by individuals preparing for workplace transitions, upgrades, or changes; pre-nursing studies; and in-house or on-the-job training programs and general brush up for work in the health care professions. The work text was designed with student success in mind. This edition includes a basic mathematics approach as well as dimensional analysis for all the application units.

The work text focuses on the needs of adult learners and features the following learner-based tools for success:

- sequential skill building on basic math skills
- ties to the application of the skill with each math concept
- mnemonic devices to build memory of the basic skills
- a variety of practice opportunities with occupation-based examples and problems
- mixed applications which build on the basic skills and promote critical thinking
- self-tests to promote confidence and skill building
- white spaces for thinking and working through the problems.

These materials have been successfully applied to help students prepare for a wide variety of health care training fields at a technical college. The student feedback and input has played a prominent role in the design and sequencing of the material, the methods of teaching, and presenting to new students. Thus, the organization of the text is central to the student's success. The students who have worked through these materials have been successful in their vocational training and workplace upgrading because they have reached a mastery level in the fundamental concepts; they are ready for the additional concepts and applications of their specific training areas.

The author has nearly 27 years of experience teaching a wide variety of adults including: second-language learners, industry experts, college preparatory students, public agency personnel, and other faculty. She embraces the attitude that all students can learn math. Furthermore, she believes that the student's success is often tied to the presentation of materials. Therefore, the colloquial quality of this text's explanation of math processes creates a can-do approach and image of math. In health care, math is a job skill, and in turn, this proficiency will promote more job opportunities.

The third edition of this work text provides a reorganization of the metric system unit so that it is placed with Roman numerals in the whole numbers unit with time in allied health. Additions to the text include, pre-algebra basics, a separate metric unit, reading drug labels, medicine cups, syringes, intravenous administration bags, parenteral dosages, basic intravenous administration, and basic dosage by weight units. Each unit has instruction, practice, and self-assessment as a structure. The context is for allied health students. This contextualization helps students appreciate the value of learning math for their careers. The unit self-tests include 15 questions, providing more practice in self-assessment. This edition has provided the odd numbers answers in the key at the end of the work text. In addition, extra practice units are included in an appendix with the answer keys for easy self-checking. The accompanying CD-ROM includes another set of practice tests with answers.

The Instructor's Resource Manual has reproducible tests that accompany the work text as a ready test bank on which instructors can rely. The unit tests (two per unit) ask the student to perform math calculations similar to those in the units. These unit tests each require 25 answers; thus the tests do not overwhelm the student, but promote self-reliance and confidence building in math.

Two post-tests are included which asks students to supply a total of 50 answers.

Reviewers

I would like to thank the reviewers of this book for their suggestions, comments, and encouragement. Their encouragement and feedback are greatly appreciated. These reviewers include:

Stacey May, AAS, CST, CSA
Director, Surgical Technology
South Plains College
Lubbock, Texas

Stacie Lynch Newberg, PhD
Assistant Professor, Developmental Studies
Western Wyoming Community College
Rock Springs, Wyoming

Vincent Range, MAT
Assistant Professor, Mathematics
Jefferson College
Hillsboro, Missouri

Rebecca Thoms, RN, CANP
Instructor
Pima Medical Institute
Tucson, Arizona

Richard L. Witt
Instructor, Pharmacy Technician Program
Allegany College of Maryland
Cumberland, Maryland

Lisa Wright, MS
Program Coordinator, Medical Assisting
Bristol Community College
Fall River, Massachusetts

Health Occupations Matrix of Math Skills and Pre-Test

Each health care field has its own emphasis and requirements for math skills. Many successful adults search out materials that serve their immediate learning needs because their studies are just one part of their busy day. This workbook has been designed to help you measure your readiness for additional math training in and for your specific field.

To assist individuals new to health occupations, a matrix of skills has been developed to answer the question: What math do I need to know to be a _____? Refer to the matrix to attain a general idea of the math skills necessary for your program preparation or workplace upgrade. These skills will form the core of your math abilities, and you will build on them in more specific ways within your specific field of study.

Once you understand what math skills are needed for your program success, you are ready to take the self-assessment. This tool is divided into categories that match the workbook's content to help you work independently or within a classroom, and it allows you to begin at your own comfort or skill level. The idea is to provide enough review and practice so that you are able to calculate the problems for your program accurately and efficiently. Use the scoring sheet to prepare an individualized study plan for yourself or as a sheet to refer to when these units are covered to ensure that you have mastered the material.

By completing this workbook, you will be ready for the specific math training that you will receive in your program of study or from the workplace.

A final word about calculators: Calculators are wonderful tools. However, calculator use may be limited to certain instances, and calculators may or may not be allowed on exams. For these reasons, mental math is a valuable skill to review. Put your calculator away as you work through these materials, and two things will result: your proficiency will increase, and your self-confidence will soar as you become an efficient math problem solver.

Matrix of Skills

	Certified nursing assistant	Hospital nursing assistant	Massage therapist	Dental assistant	Pharmacy technician	Surgical technologist	Medical assistant	Licensed practical nurse	Registered nurse	Medical lab technician	Your program		
Practice Pre-test	X	X	X	X	X	X	X	X	X	X			
Unit 1: Whole number review	X	X	X	X	X	X	X	X	X	X			
Unit 2: Fractions	X	X	X	X	X	X	X	X	X	X			
Unit 3: Decimals	X	X	X	X	X	X	X	X	X	X			
Unit 4: Ratio and proportion	X	X	X	X	X	X	X	X	X	X			
Unit 5: Percents	X	X	X	X	X	X	X	X	X	X			
Unit 6: Combined applications	X	X	X	X	X	X	X	X	X	X			
Unit 7: Pre-algebra basics	X	X	X	X	X	X	X	X	X	X			
Unit 8: The metric system	X	X	X	X	X	X	X	X	X				
Unit 9: Reading drug labels, medicine cups, syringes, and intravenous fluid administration bags	X	X	X	X	X	X	X	X	X	X			
Unit 10: Apothecary measurement and conversion					X		X	X	X				
Unit 11: Dosage calculation					X		X	X	X				
Unit 12: Parenteral dosage					X		X	X	X				
Unit 13: The basics of intravenous fluid administration					X		X	X	X				
Unit 14: Basic dosage by weight					X		X	X	X				
Practice Post-test	X	X	X	X	X	X	X	X	X	X			

The Math for Health Care Professionals Pre-Test is provided on the next several pages. The pre-test is designed to highlight the major points in each of the fourteen units. Some of these skills may be review while others may be new topics to study.

Math for Health Care Professionals Pre-Test

Whole Number Skills

1. Find the mean of the set of numbers: 16, 10, 5, 9, 10, 7, 3, 20
    _____

2. 609 + _____ + 37 = 812

3. 1876 − 618 = _____

4. 34 × 97 = _____

5. $26\overline{)324}$ = _____

6. The heights of the members of Michele's family are 67 inches, 81 inches, 69 inches, 70 inches, and 68 inches. Find the range in height of the members of Michele's family. _____

7. Convert from 3:15 P.M. standard time to universal time. _____

Fraction Skills

8. Order the fractions from smallest to largest: $\frac{7}{8}, \frac{5}{6}, \frac{1}{4}, \frac{3}{4}$ _____

9. $30\frac{3}{5} + 12 + 3\frac{5}{6} =$ _____

10. $46\frac{1}{3} - 8\frac{7}{12} =$ _____

11. $3\frac{4}{5} \times \frac{3}{7} \times 5 =$ _____

12. $7\frac{1}{6} \div \frac{1}{2} =$ _____

13. Solve: $\dfrac{\frac{1}{20}}{\frac{1}{4}} =$ _____

Decimal Skills

14. Express as a fraction: 8.022 _____

15. Express as a decimal: $6\frac{7}{8}$ _____

16. $10.6 + 0.5 + 9 =$ _____

17. $59.3 - 5.65 =$ _____

18. $0.6 \times 31.2 =$ _____

19. $228.06 \div 0.4 =$ _____

Ratio and Proportion Skills

20. A container holds 54 milliliters of medication. How many full 1.25 milliliter doses can be administered from this container? _____

21. Solve: $6 : 75 :: 2.5 : x$ $x =$ _____

22. Solve: $7 : x :: 42 : 200$

    $x =$ _____ Write the answer as a mixed number.

23. Solve: $\frac{1}{4} : 8 :: x : 72$ $x =$ _____

24. Solve: $\frac{1}{50} : 5 :: \frac{10}{250} : x$ $x =$ _____

25. Simplify the ratio to the lowest terms: $2\frac{1}{2} : 3$ _____

Percent Skills

26. What is $11\frac{3}{4}\%$ of 55? _____ Round to the nearest tenth.

27. What percent is 22 of 144? _____ Round to the nearest hundredth.

28. 16% of 140 is what number? _____

29. The original price of a new nursing jacket is $42.50. There is a 15% discount. What is the new price for the nursing jacket before tax? Round the discounted amount, then calculate the discount.

    _____

30. There are 5 grams of pure drug are in 65 mL of solution. What is the percent strength of solution? _____

Combined Application

31. $3\frac{1}{4}$ feet = _____ inches

32. _____ quarts = 12 pints

33. 15 pounds = _____ kilograms

34. _____ teaspoons = 30 milliliters

35. Convert 0.5% to a fraction = _____

36. Convert $3\frac{1}{2}$ to a percent = _____

37. Convert 18 to a percent = _____

38. Write 1.001 as a fraction = _____

39. Write 0.07% as a decimal = _____

Pre-Algebra

40. $45 + (-10) =$ _____

41. $-12 - 42 =$ _____

42. $-63 \div 9 =$ _____

43. $-128 \times (-4) =$ _____

44. $32 + \sqrt{144} =$ _____

45. $(5^2 - 3^2) \div 5 =$ _____

Metric Measurements

46. 129.45 micrograms = _____ milligrams

47. 94 grams = _____ kilogram Round to the nearest tenth.

48. Complete the table for this drug label. If the information is not provided, write *Not shown.*

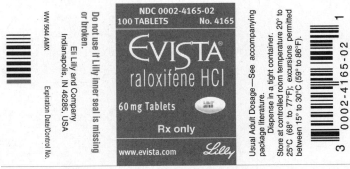

Generic name   _____

Trade name   _____

Manufacturer   _____

National Drug Code (NDC) number   _____

Lot number (control number)   _____

Drug form   _____

Dosage strength   _____

Usual adult dose   _____

Total amount in vial, packet, box   _____

Prescription warning   _____

Expiration date   _____

49. The medical assistant was asked to dispense 14 milliliters of a liquid medication. Shade the medicine cup to indicate this dosage.

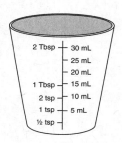

50. The physician has ordered an intramuscular (IM) injection of 1.8 milliliters. Shade the syringe to indicate this volume of medication.

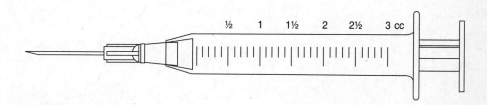

Apothecary Measurements

51. fluid ounces 18 = _____ milliliters

52. 16 teaspoons = _____ milliliters

53. 3 pints = _____ milliliters

54. 0.5 milligrams = grain _____

55. grain $\frac{1}{300}$ = _____ milligrams

56. 3 grams = grains _____

57. $3\frac{1}{2}$ teaspoons = _____ milliliters

Oral Medications

58. Desired: Aspirin 1.5 grams every 4 hours
    Available: Aspirin 500 milligrams scored tablets
    Give: _____

59. The patient is prescribed Vistaril 20 milligrams orally every 6 hours for nausea relief. You have on hand Vistaril oral suspension 5 milligrams in 2.5 milliliters.
    You adminster _____.

Dosage Calculations

60. Ordered: Zocor 40 milligrams
    Have: Zocar 20 milligrams per tablet
    Give: _____

61. The doctor has ordered Zyloprim 0.25 gram orally twice a day. On hand is Zyloprim 100 milligrams scored tablets. The nurse should give _____.

62. The client receives an order for Augmentin 250 milligrams. The Augmentin is labeled 125 milligrams in 5 milliliter. The client will be given _____.

Parenteral Dosages

63. The physician orders megestrol acetate 800 milligrams per day. The megestrol acetate label reads oral suspension 40 milligrams per milliliter. Give _____.

64. Give Dilaudid 0.5 milligram. IM from a vial that is labeled 4 milligrams per milliliter. Give _____. Round to the nearest hundredth.

65. Ordered: Atropine sulfate 0.5 milligram IM
    Have: Atropine sulfate 0.3 milligram per milliliter
    Give   _____. Round to the nearest hundredth.

66. The doctor prescribes heparin 3500 units sub-Q four times a day. You have heparin 2500 units per milliliter. You give _____.

67. Ordered: quinidine 0.4 grams orally every 4 hours. Quinidine is supplied in 200 milligrams tablets. How many tablets will you give?
    _____

Calculating IV Dosages

68. The patient with oliguria has an order for 75 milliliters of 0.9% normal saline (NS) over 2 hours. The drop factor is 15 drops per milliliter (gtt/mL). How many drops per minute should be given? _____

69. The nurse receives an order that reads 1200 milliliters 5% dextrose water (D_5W) intravenous (IV) at 150 milliliters per hour. Infuse for _____.

70. The nurse will administer an IV solution at 115 milliliters per hour for 12 hours. What is the total volume infused? _____

Basic Dosages by Body Weight

Do the calculations to determine whether the following prescription is a therapeutic dosage for this child:

    Ordered medication ABC 5 milligrams orally every 12 hours for a child weighing 14 pounds. You have medication ABC 15 milligrams per milliliter. The recommended daily oral dosage for a child is 2.5 milligrams per kilogram per day in divided doses every 12 hours.

> **Medication ABC**
> **Oral Solution**
> 15 mg/mL

71. This child's weight is _____ kilograms.

72. What is the recommended dosage for this child? _____ milligrams per day

Weight: 34 pounds 6 ounces
Ordered dosage: 1.4 milligrams per kilogram per day
Recommended dosage from drug label: 3 milligrams every 8 hours

73. What is the daily dose? _____

74. What is the individual dose? _____

75. Does the ordered dose match the recommended dosage? _____

Answers

1. 10

2. 166

3. 1258

4. 3298

5. 12.46 or 12 R 12 or $12\frac{6}{13}$

6. 14

7. 1515

8. $\frac{1}{4}, \frac{3}{4}, \frac{5}{6}, \frac{7}{8}$

9. $46\frac{13}{30}$

10. $37\frac{3}{4}$

11. $8\frac{1}{7}$

12. $14\frac{1}{3}$, 14 R 1, 14.33

13. $\frac{1}{5}$

14. $8\frac{11}{500}$

15. 6.875

16. 20.1

17. 53.65

18. 18.72

19. 570.15

20. 43.2

21. 31.25

22. $33\frac{1}{3}$

23. 2.25

24. 10

25. 5 : 6

26. 6.5

27. 15.28

28. 22.40

29. $36.12

30. 7.7%

31. 39

32. 6

33. 6.8

34. 6

35. $\frac{1}{200}$

36. 350%

37. 1800%

38. $1\frac{1}{1000}$

39. 0.007

40. 35

41. −54

42. −7

43. 512

44. 44

45. 3.2 or $3\frac{1}{5}$

46. 0.12945

47. 0.1

48. Generic name   Raloxifene HCl

     Trade name   Evista

     Manufacturer   Eli Lily and Company

     National Drug Code (NDC) number   0002-4165-02

     Lot number (control number)   Not shown

     Drug form   Tablets

     Dosage strength   60 milligrams

     Usual adult dose   Not shown; see accompanying
                                           package literature

     Total amount in vial, packet, box   100 tablets

     Prescription warning   Rx only

     Expiration date   Not shown

49. 14 milliliters of a liquid medication.

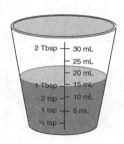

50. 1.8 milliliters Shade the syringe to indicate this volume of medication.

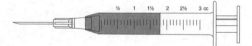

51. 540 milliliters

52. 80 milliliters

53. 1500 milliliters

54. grain $\frac{1}{200}$

55. 0.2 milligram

56. grains 50

57. 17.5 milliliters

58. 3 tablets

59. 10 milliliters

60. 2 tablets

61. $2\frac{1}{2}$ tablets

62. 10 milliliters

63. 20 milliliters

64. 0.13 milliliter

65. 1.67 milliliters

66. 1.4 milliliters

67. 2 tablets

68. 9 drops per minute

69. 8 hours

70. 1380 milliliters

71. 6.36 kilograms

72. 15.9 milligrams per day

73. 21.88 milligrams per day

74. 7.29 milligrams per dose

75. No, contact physician for clarification.

Unit 1

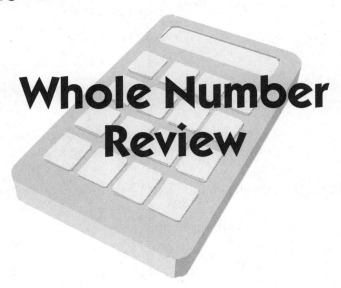

Whole Number Review

Mathematics is a key skill of health care workers. As a health care worker, you know that accuracy is important. Being competent in whole number concepts and addition, subtraction, multiplication, and division will form the basis for successful computations on the job. These basic skills form the foundation for the other daily math functions you will use in the workplace.

> Approach math matter-of-factly; math is a job skill and a life skill.

The number line is a line labeled with the integers in increasing order from left to right. The number line extends in both directions:

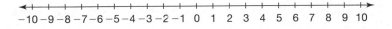

$$-10\ -9\ -8\ -7\ -6\ -5\ -4\ -3\ -2\ -1\quad 0\quad 1\quad 2\quad 3\quad 4\quad 5\quad 6\quad 7\quad 8\quad 9\quad 10$$

Remember that any integer on the right is always greater than the integer on the left.

Symbols and Number Statements

Symbols may be used to show the relationship among numbers.

Symbol	Meaning	Example
=	is equal to	$1 + 7 = 8$
>	is greater than	$19 > 6$
<	is less than	$5 < 12$
≤	is equal to or less than	age ≤ 5
≥	is equal to or greater than	weight ≥ 110 pounds

A number statement or simple equation shows the relationship between numbers, operations and/or symbols.

Practice 1: Use the symbols (=, >, and <, ≤, ≥) to complete the number statement.

1. 14 _____ 34
2. −5 _____ 0
3. 12 _____ 7
4. 12 P.M. _____ noon
5. Seven less than 4 _____ the numbers −5, −4, −3
6. $2.00 _____ 2 hundred pennies
7. 235 _____ 187
8. 2 nickels _____ a quarter
9. 245 _____ 78 + 34 + 3
10. One dollar + 2 quarters _____ $1.35
11. The numbers 0, 1, 2, are _____ the number 2
12. 3 _____ 4 ÷ 2

Practice 2: Write five number statements:

1. _____
2. _____
3. _____
4. _____
5. _____

Addition

Review

To add, line up the numbers in a vertical column and add to find the total. In addition problems, the total, or answer, is called the *sum*.

Practice Find the sum of each problem.

1. $1 + 4 + 5 + 9 =$
2. $51 + 23 =$
3. $297 + 90 + 102 + 3 =$
4. $216 + 897 =$
5. $1,773 + 233 + 57 =$
6. $9 + 245 + 32 =$
7. $11 + 357 + 86 + 34 =$
8. $24,578 + 9,075 =$
9. $443 + 2,087 + 134 =$
10. $910 + 3 + 125 =$

Applications Inventory is an important clerical function in the health care industry. Sometimes this work is done by supply technicians, clerks, nursing assistants, or other staff. Keeping accurate inventory reduces overstocking and helps avoid the problem of under stocking medical supplies.

1. Inventory is done monthly at the Golden Years Care Center. Find the sum for each category.

Category	Sum
a. Examination gloves: $31 + 88 + 47 +$ two boxes of 50	_____
b. Thermometer covers: $281 + 304 + 17 + 109$	_____
c. Medicine cups: $313 + 245 + 106 + 500 + 12$	_____
d. Boxes of disposable syringes (50 per box): $2 + 6 + 9 + 3$	_____

2. Intake and output totals require addition skills. Unlike household measurements in cups, health care patient intake and output units are measured in cubic centimeters (cc). Intake includes oral ingestion of fluids and semi-liquid food, intravenous feedings, and tubal feedings.
   Find the intake totals.

Type of Intake	Cubic Centimeters (cc)	Sum
a. Oral	120, 210, 150, 240	_____
b. Intravenous	250, 500	_____
c. Blood	500	_____
d.	Total Intake	_____

The intake sums would be charted in the patient's medical record.

3. Measuring output is important because it helps the health care worker ensure a patient's health and hydration. Output is measured in cubic

centimeters. Output includes liquid bowel movements or diarrhea, urine, emesis (vomiting), and gastric drainage. Find the output totals.

	Type of Output	Cubic Centimeters (cc)	Sum
a.	Diarrhea	100, 200	____
b.	Urine	330, 225, 105, 60	____
c.	Gastric Drainage	40, 35	____
d.	Blood/Emesis	110	____
e.		Total Output	____

4. Assuming that the patient is the same as in problems 2 and 3, has this patient had a greater intake or a greater output? _____

Subtraction

Review

To subtract, line up the numbers according to place value. Place value shows the ones, tens, hundreds, etc. columns. Start with the right side of the math problem and work your way toward the left side, subtracting each column.

> Fewer errors occur if the subtraction problem is set up vertically. Rewrite the problems.

Example

$$89 - 31 = \underline{\qquad} \qquad\qquad 475 - 34 = \underline{\qquad}$$

$$\begin{array}{r} 89 \\ -31 \\ \hline 58 \end{array} \qquad\qquad \begin{array}{r} 475 \\ -34 \\ \hline 441 \end{array}$$

If a number cannot be subtracted from the number directly above it, then increase the value of the smaller number by borrowing 1 from the column to its immediate left.

> Keep track of borrowing by marking through the column borrowed from and reducing the numbers involved by 1.

Example

$$\begin{array}{r} 3^7\cancel{8}^11 \\ -\ 65 \\ \hline 316 \end{array}$$

Practice
1. $475 - 81 =$
2. $176 - 37 =$
3. $289 - 54 =$
4. $4,547 - 2,289 =$
5. $1,236 - 799 =$
6. $1,575 - 896 =$
7. $2,001 - 128 =$
8. $10,300 - 497 =$
9. $4,301 - 89 =$
10. $4,547 - 2,289 =$

Applications   Subtraction is used in inventory as well. Some applications are given below.

1. At the beginning of the month, a dental office started with 2,258 latex examination gloves. On the last working day of the month, 784 remained. How many gloves were used during the month?

2. Inventory of dental file labels is to be kept at 2,000. Paula's inventory indicates 579 on hand. How many labels does she need to order?

3. Labels come in boxes of 500. Use the answer from problem 2 to determine how many boxes of labels Paula should order to obtain the required 2,000 minimum inventory. Draw a sketch to help visualize this problem.

4. Patients see the dentist most during the summer months. Dr. Brown has a total of 13,576 patient files. If he sees 8,768 of these patients during the summer, how many remain to be contacted for an appointment?

Multiplication

Memorizing the multiplication tables is essential to sound mental math. If you have been calculator dependent or have forgotten some of the tables, practice memorizing the multiplication tables using the chart shown in Table 1.1.

Table 1.1   Multiplication Table

X	1	2	3	4	5	6	7	8	9	10	11	12
1												
2												
3												
4												
5												
6												
7												
8												
9												
10												
11												
12												

Review

To multiply, line up the numbers according to place value. By putting the largest number on top of the problem, you will avoid careless errors.

Avoid These Common Errors

Remember, you are multiplying, not adding.

Remember to move the numbers from the second and succeeding lines over one column to the left—use a zero (0) to indicate these movements.

$$2 \times 14 = \underline{\hspace{1cm}} \qquad \rightarrow \begin{array}{r} 14 \\ \times\ 2 \\ \hline 28 \end{array}$$

$$\begin{array}{r} 178 \\ \times\quad 23 \\ \hline 534 \\ 3560 \\ \hline 4{,}094 \end{array}$$

Move the second line of numbers one place to the left. Adding a zero keeps your numbers aligned.

Practice

1. $\begin{array}{r} 12 \\ \times\ 8 \\ \hline \end{array}$	4. $\begin{array}{r} 70 \\ \times\ 9 \\ \hline \end{array}$	7. $\begin{array}{r} 512 \\ \times\ 24 \\ \hline \end{array}$	10. $\begin{array}{r} 803 \\ \times\ 17 \\ \hline \end{array}$
2. $\begin{array}{r} 82 \\ \times\ 13 \\ \hline \end{array}$	5. $\begin{array}{r} 1,020 \\ \times\ 98 \\ \hline \end{array}$	8. $\begin{array}{r} 927 \\ \times\ 35 \\ \hline \end{array}$	11. $\begin{array}{r} 346 \\ \times\ 12 \\ \hline \end{array}$
3. $\begin{array}{r} 1,306 \\ \times\ 18 \\ \hline \end{array}$	6. $\begin{array}{r} 189 \\ \times\ 27 \\ \hline \end{array}$	9. $\begin{array}{r} 5,791 \\ \times\ 16 \\ \hline \end{array}$	12. $\begin{array}{r} 9,004 \\ \times\ 73 \\ \hline \end{array}$

Applications

1. Last month a nurse worked fourteen 10-hour shifts and two 12-hour shifts. At $21 per hour, what was the nurse's total hourly income before deductions?

2. Health-care facilities monitor all medications taken by their patients. Assume that the same dosage is given each time the medication is dispensed. What is the total daily dosage of each medication received?

   Total medication received is as follows:

   a. Patient Bao   50 milligrams   4 times a day   _____ milligrams

   b. Patient Mary   25 milligrams   2 times a day   _____ milligrams

   c. Patient Luke   125 micrograms   3 times a day   _____ micrograms

   d. Patient Vang   375 micrograms   2 times a day   _____ micrograms

3. The radiology lab ordered 15 jackets for its staff. The jackets cost approximately $35 each. What is the estimated cost of this order?

Prime Factorization

Sometimes in a math class, students are asked to use factor trees to illustrate prime factors of a number. A factor is a number which divides exactly into another number. When two or more factors are multiplied, they form a product. A prime factor is a number that can only be the product of 1 and itself.

For example: 4 (factor) $\times$ 12 (factor) = 48 (product)

The prime factors of 48 are 2 and 3.
($2 \times 2 \times 2 \times 3 = 24$)

$$
\begin{array}{c}
48 \\
\wedge \\
4 \quad 12 \\
\wedge \quad \wedge \\
2\ 2 \quad 4\ 3 \\
\wedge \\
2\ 2
\end{array}
$$

$2 \times 2 \times 2 \times 2 \times 3 = \mathbf{48}$
or $\ 2^4 \cdot 3 = \mathbf{48}$
or $\ (2^4)(3) = \mathbf{48}$

Note that $16 \times 3 = 48$.

The prime factors are still the same:

$2 \times 2 \times 2 \times 2 \times 3$.

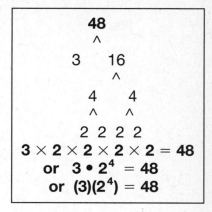

The prime factors are always the same for any number.

Practice   Draw the factor trees for the following numbers and write the prime factors on the lines below.

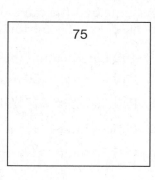   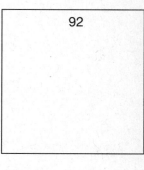

124	75	92

1. _____   2. _____   3. _____

Division

Review

To divide whole numbers determine (a) what number is being divided into smaller portions; and (b) the size of the portions.

Division can appear in three formats:

  a. $27 \div 3 =$

  b. Twenty-seven divided by three

  c. $3\overline{)27}$

Setting up the problem correctly will help ensure the correct answer.

Example

$$81 \quad \div \quad 3 = \text{\_\_\_\_\_}$$
$$\uparrow \qquad\quad \uparrow$$
$$\text{dividend} \quad \text{divisor}$$

means eighty-one divided by three or how many 3s are in 81. The answer is the quotient.

$$27 \leftarrow \text{quotient}$$
$$\text{divisor} \rightarrow 3\overline{)81} \leftarrow \text{dividend}$$
$$\underline{6}$$
$$21$$
$$\underline{21}$$
$$0$$

Practice the correct setup, but do not work the problems.

1. Divide 145 by 76

2. $1{,}209 \div 563$

3. Forty-nine divided by seventeen is what number?

4. What is $8{,}794 \div 42$?

5. A person works a total of 2,044 hours a year. How many days does the person work if he works 8 hours a day?

Follow the steps below to complete all of your whole number division problems:

Step 1: Underline the number of places that the divisor can go into, then write the number of times the divisor can go into the dividend on the quotient line. Place it directly above the underlined portion of the number. This keeps track of your process. Multiply the number by the divisor and place it below the underlined portion of the dividend. Then subtract the numbers.

Example

$$1$$
$$34\overline{)5492}$$
$$\underline{-34}$$
$$20$$

Step 2: Bring down the next number of the dividend. Use an arrow to keep alignment and track of which numbers you have worked with. Then repeat step 1.

$$161$$
$$34\overline{)5492}$$
$$\underline{-34\downarrow}$$
$$20$$

$$161 \text{ R } 18$$
$$34\overline{)5492}$$
$$\underline{-34\downarrow}$$
$$209$$
$$\underline{204\downarrow}$$
$$52$$
$$\underline{34}$$
$$18$$

Repeat steps 1 and 2 until all the numbers of the dividend have been used. The number remaining is called the remainder. Place it next to an *R* to the right of the quotient. In fractions, the remainder becomes a fraction; in whole numbers, it remains a whole number.

After bringing a number down from the dividend, a number must be placed in the quotient. Zeros may be used as place holders. Follow the division steps as shown above to solve the practice problems.

$$
\begin{array}{r}
106 \text{ R } 41 \\
75\overline{)7991} \\
-75\downarrow \\
\hline
49 \\
-0\downarrow \\
\hline
491 \\
-450 \\
\hline
41
\end{array}
$$

Practice

1. $6\overline{)564}$

2. $3\overline{)5736}$

3. $4\overline{)12345}$

4. $956 \div 66 =$

5. $4\overline{)1244}$

6. $53\overline{)5088}$

7. $15\overline{)23648}$

8. $1{,}254 \div 29 =$

9. $2\overline{)46882}$

10. $18\overline{)12564}$

11. $7\overline{)87543}$

12. $74{,}943 \div 271 =$

Applications

1. Room rates vary by the services provided. At the local hospital, intensive care unit (ICU) rooms are $784 a day. Bob's overall room charge was $10,192. How many days was Bob in ICU?

2. Carbohydrates have 4 calories per gram. If a serving of soup has 248 calories of carbohydrates, how many grams of carbohydrates are in that serving?

3. A medical assistant subscribes to 14 magazines for the office. If the total subscription bill is $294, what is the average cost of each magazine subscription?

4. A pharmacy technician receives a shipment of 302 boxes of acetamino-phen. This shipment needs to be returned to the supplier because the expiration date on the medicine did not allow sufficient time to sell the medicine. If each case holds 36 individual boxes, how many cases must the pharmacy technician use to pack the medicine?

5. A surgical technologist made $39,744 last year. He is paid twice a month. What is the gross or total amount of each of his paychecks?

6. A licensed practical nurse gives 1,800 milligrams of a penicillin-type drug over a 36-hour time period. If the dosage occurs every 6 hours, how many milligrams are in each dose if each dose is the same amount?

7. Each gram of fat contains 9 calories. How many grams of fat are in 81 calories of fat in a piece of steak?

Solving for the Unknown Number with Basic Mathematics

Sometimes number statements in math class ask for the unknown number. Looking for an unknown number is an aspect of algebra. Solving for these requires that one understand the relationship between the numbers.

For example, _____ $+ 12 = 75$

To find the unknown number, you must subtract 12 from 75. The answer, or unknown number, is 63.

Practice 1:   Use addition to solve for the unknown number.

1. $13 +$ _____ $= 87$

2. _____ $+ 12 + 2 = 145$

3. $45 +$ _____ $= 98$

4. _____ $= 98 + 17$

5. _____ $+ 987 = 1,000$

Practice 2:   Use subtraction to solve for the unknown number.

1. $98 - 12 =$ _____

2. $237 -$ _____ $= 67$

3. _____ $- 17 = 543$

4. $45 - 19 =$ _____

5. $12 =$ _____ $- 23$

Practice 3:   Use multiplication to solve for the unknown number.

1. $13 \times 3 =$ _____

2. _____ $\times 11 = 99$

3. _____ $\times 23 = 92$

4. $125 \times$ _____ $= 500$

5. _____ $= 15 \times 5$

Practice 4:   Use division to solve for the unknown number.

1. $396 \div 3 =$ _____

2. _____ $\div 12 = 4$

3. $51 \div$ _____ $= 17$

4. $125 =$ _____ $\div 5$

5. $108 \div 6 =$ _____

Rounding

Review

Whole numbers have place values. The number 3,195 has four specific place values: $\dfrac{3, \quad 1 \quad 9 \quad 5}{\uparrow \quad \uparrow \quad \uparrow \quad \uparrow}$ (three thousand one hundred ninety-five)

thousand hundreds tens ones

By using the place values in a number, we can round the number to a particular and specific place unit. Rounding is valuable because it helps to estimate supplies, inventory, and countable items to the nearest unit.

> Rounding is used when an exact number is not necessary, as in taking inventory and ordering: Round up to make a full case of a product when you are placing an order. If a full case has 36 boxes and you need to order 32 boxes, you will order 1 case or 36 boxes, so you have rounded up to the nearest case.

Rounding is accomplished in three steps.

Example Round 7,872 to the nearest hundred.

Step 1: Locate the hundreds place and underline it.

7,872

Step 2: Circle the number to the right of the underlined number.

7,8⑦2

Step 3: If the circled number is 5 or greater, add 1 to the underlined number and change the number(s) to the right of the underlined number to zero(s).

7, 8 ⑦ 2
     ↓ ↓
7, 9 0 0

Rounding is used a great deal in health care. Rounding of whole numbers exists in inventory and packaging of supplies as well as in daily activities.

Practice 1. Round to the nearest 10:

    a. 3,918 _____ c. 6,952 _____ e. 15,932 _____

    b. 139 _____ d. 1,925 _____ f. 99 _____

2. Round to the nearest 100:

    a. 3,918 _____ c. 8,975 _____ e. 35,292 _____

    b. 3,784 _____ d. 17,854 _____ f. 1,925 _____

3. Round to the nearest 1,000:

    a. 3,190 _____ c. 6,950 _____ e. 432,500 _____

    b. 87,987 _____ d. 12,932 _____ f. 2,987 _____

Additional rounding practice will be presented in Unit 3: Decimals.

Estimation

Estimation is a method of coming up with a math answer that is general, not specific. When we estimate, we rely on rounding to help us get to this general answer. For example, with money rounding is done to the nearest dollar. If an amount has 50 cents or more, *round* to the nearest dollar and drop the cent amount. If an amount is under 50 cents, *retain* the dollar amount and drop the cent amount.

Example   Estimate Bob's expenses for his co-payment of his dental expenses for his two six-month checkups.

	Actual Expense	Estimated Expense
March	$65.85	$66
October	$59.10	$59

Add the estimated expenses of $66 + $59 = _____
The estimated annual total is $125.
So estimation is a skill that uses rounding to reach a general rather than a specific answer.

Practice   1. Find the sum using estimation to the nearest dollar:
   a. $56.90 + $12.45 + $124.78
   b. $127.46 + $13.98 + $21.20
   c. $23.45 + $32.29 + $56.65
   d. $2,900.87 + $12.89

2. Find the sum using estimation to the nearest hour:
   a. 1 hour 25 minutes + 2 hours 14 minutes + 5 hours 37 minutes
   b. 7 hours 8 minutes + 10 hours 34 minutes + 15 hours 45 minutes
   c. 3 hours 35 minutes + 22 hours 16 minutes + 9 hours 59 minutes
   d. 6 hours 39 minutes + 13 hours 18 minutes + 5 hours 2 minutes

Basics of Statistical Analysis

The basics of statistical analysis includes the topics of *mean* (average), *mode*, *median*, and *range*. Each of these topics deals with groups or subsets of numbers and their relationships to each other and the set as a whole.

Arithmetic Mean or Average

Review   The arithmetic *mean* is also called the average. An average is a number that represents a group of the same unit of measure. It provides a general number that represents this group of numbers if all the numbers were the same units. Averages are useful in health occupations because they provide general trends and information. Averages are computed using addition and division skills.
   To compute a mean or average, follow these two steps:

Step 1:   Add the individual units of measure.

Step 2:   Divide the sum of the units of measure by the number of individual units.

Example   Mary Ann wanted to know the average score of her anatomy and physiology tests. Her scores were 92%, 79%, 100%, 89%, and 95%.

Step 1: $92 + 79 + 100 + 89 + 95 = 455$

Step 2: There were a total of 5 grades.

Mary Ann's average score was 91%.

$$
\begin{array}{r}
91 \\
5\overline{)455} \\
45\downarrow \\
\hline
5 \\
5 \\
\hline
0
\end{array}
$$

Practice

1. Deb needed to purchase new calendars for the examination rooms. Find the average if the calendars cost $11, $7, $10, $5, $10, $12, $8, and $9.

2. Certified nursing assistants work a varied number of hours every week at Village Nursing Home. The weekly hours are 32, 38, 40, 35, 40, 16, and 30. What is the average number of hours each assistant works?

3. The staff phone use during morning break is increasing. The director is considering adding additional phones and is researching the usage in minutes. Using the following data, compute the average length of each call: 7, 4, 3, 1, 2, 4, 5, 7, and 12.

4. A diabetic patient is counting calories. The patient adds up calories from portions of fruit: 90, 80, 60, 15, 40. What is the average caloric intake from each portion?

5. Beth was working hard to increase the fruit and vegetables in her diet. She kept a log of servings: Monday, 8; Tuesday, 7; Wednesday, 6; Thursday, 5; Friday, 8; Saturday, 6; Sunday, 9. What is the mean daily intake of fruits and vegetables for Beth?

Median

The *median* is the middle number in a list of numbers. To determine the median, follow these steps:

Step 1: Sort the list of numbers from smallest to largest.

Step 2: Cross off one number from each end of the line of numbers until one number is reached in the middle.

Example   Find the median of this set of numbers: 23, 54, 76, 34, 12.

Step 1: Sort from smallest to largest   12, 23, 34, 54, 76

Step 2: Cross a number off from each end   ~~12~~, 23, 34, 54, ~~76~~
until the middle number is reached.   ~~12~~, ~~23~~, 34, ~~54~~, ~~76~~

34 is the median

If there is an even set of numbers, the final two numbers are added and then divided by 2 to get the median. For example, consider the following set of numbers: 23, 54, 76, 34, 12, 36.

Step 1: Sort from smallest to largest   12, 23, 34, 36, 54, 76

Step 2: Cross a number off from each end   ~~12~~, 23, 34, 36, 54, ~~76~~
until the last pair is reached.   ~~12~~, ~~23~~, 34, 36, ~~54~~, ~~76~~

Step 3: Add the two remaining numbers   34 + 36 = 70

Step 4: Divide the answer by 2 to get the   70 ÷ 2 = 35
median.

35 is the median.

Note: The median may include a partial number such as $\frac{1}{2}$ or 0.5.

Practice   1. Bah's temperature fluctuated all day. Her temperature readings were 98, 99, 97, 101, and 100. What is her median temperature?

2. The young patients played a game. The scores for five games were 365, 251, 105, 280, and 198. What is the median of this set of scores?

3. The medical assistant was working on inventory. She wanted to figure out the median of the number of cases of protective sheeting that were used for the first six months of the year in the large medical practice.

Month	Number of cases
January	26
February	22
March	31
April	28
May	26
June	19

What is the median for this set of data?

4. Azeb is an excellent student. She is curious about the median of her test scores in biology class. Her scores are 99, 100, 98, 97, 100. Her median is _____.

5. The students were measuring tardiness to class by incidence each week. Look at the data set: 7, 8, 10, 10, 15, 12, 8, 7. What is the mean of this data set?

Mode

The mode is the "most popular" value or the most frequently occurring item in a set of numbers to locate the mode in a series or listing of numbers, locate the number, which occurs the most.

For example, look at the calories of Bob's snack food intake for a two-day period:

Bob's caloric intake of snacks by day

Saturday: 120, 120, 50, 78, 134, 187

Sunday: 220, 125, 90, 85, 120, 120

What is the mode of the calorie intake of Bob's snack intake over this two-day period?

The answer is 120. It occurs four times.

Practice

1. Look at the pH values of the following data set: 8, 11, 23, 14, 8, 12. What is the mode for this data set?

2. Look at the prices of toothbrushes: $2.00; $4.00, $3.00; $3.00, $1.00; $3.00. What is the mode of these toothbrush prices?

3. The color combinations preferred by new dental offices include: paint sample #24, paint sample #154, paint sample #654, paint sample #24, paint sample #154, paint sample #24, and paint sample #63. What is the mode?

4. Designer eyeglass frames cost a lot. This season's top selling frame prices are from $330, $199, $230, $400, $497, and $330. What is the mode of these eyeglass frame prices?

5. The Healthville Residence is having a problem with absenteeism during the summer months.

The administrator wants to find out who is missing work the most. First add the days absent for each employee, and write the number in the "Total days absent" column. Compare the total days absent from work; what is the mode for the number of days absent for the summer months?

Employee	Days absent in June	Days absent in July	Days absent in August	Total days absent
Verna	3	2	2	_____
Xuyen	4	4	3	_____
Cam	3	2	1	_____
Debbie	3	3	3	_____
Ed	2	2	2	_____
Vasily	1	3	4	_____
Ted	3	2	2	_____

Range

The range of a set of numbers is the largest value in the set minus the smallest value in the set. Note that the range is a single number, not many numbers. The range is the difference between the largest and the smallest numbers.

For example, the hospital delivered six babies today. The weight in pounds of these newborns was 6, 9, 10, 8, 7, 5.

Step 1: Locate the smallest number and the largest number   5 and 10

Step 2: Subtract the smallest number from the largest number. $10 - 5 = 5$

The range is 5.

Practice:

1. The age of patients in the hospital fluctuates. Look at the data and calculate the range of patients' ages: 68, 94, 23, 45, 98, 100, 69 18, 25, 75, 87.

2. The workforce at the Village care Center is diverse in age. Look at the data and calculate the range of workers' ages: 19, 21, 24, 23, 45, 34, 28, 25, 31, 56, 64, 71, 49, 52.

3. The breakfast meals served in the cafeteria vary in calories. Look at the data and calculate the range of calories in the meals: 120, 220, 280, 340, 440, 480.

4. The public health nurse has a rural route to drive each week. What is the range that the daily miles, 7, 14, 23, 24, 16, 12, record?

5. The bandages sold in a local drug store have a wide price range. Each bandage costs as follows: 50 cents, 35 cents, 78 cents, 89 cents, 99 cents, 12 cents, and 25 cents. What is the range in individual bandage costs?

Roman Numerals

In our daily lives, we use Arabic numerals 0 to 9 and combinations of these digits to do most of our mathematical activities. In the health care field, Roman numerals are sometimes used along with Arabic numerals. Roman numerals are often found in prescriptions and in medical records and charts. Roman numerals consist of lower- and uppercase letters that represent numbers. For medical applications, Roman numerals will be written in lowercase letters for the numbers 1 to 10. Use uppercase when smaller numbers are part of a number over 30 such as 60: LX not lx. Do not use commas in Roman numerals.

Roman Numerals

Roman numerals are formed by combining the numbers.			
	1 = i or I	6 = vi or VI	$\frac{1}{2}$ = ss
	2 = ii or II	7 = vii or VII	50 = L
	3 = iii or III	8 = viii or VIII	100 = C
	4 = iv or IV	9 = ix or IX	500 = D
	5 = v or V	10 = x or X	1,000 = M

Mnemonic Device Note the pattern: 50-100-500-1000

L = 50	Lovely
C = 100	Cats
D = 500	Don't
M = 1000	Meow!

This will help you to remember the order and value of each Roman numeral.

Use the following basic Roman numeral concepts to accurately read and write Roman numerals.

Concept 1

Add Roman numerals of the same or decreasing value when they are placed next to each other. Read these from left to right.

Examples

$$vii = 5 + 2 = 7 \qquad\qquad xxi = 10 + 10 + 1 = 21$$

Practice Write the numerals in Arabic or Roman numerals.

1. xiii   6. 17

2. xv   7. 31

3. xxxi   8. 120

4. LV   9. $1\frac{1}{2}$

5. MI   10. 11

Concept 2

Subtract a numeral of decreasing or lesser value from the numeral to its right.

Examples

$$iv = 5 - 1 = 4 \qquad\qquad XC = 100 - 10 = 90$$

$$IM = 1000 - 1 = 999 \qquad\qquad xix = 10 + 10 - 1 = 19$$

Practice Write the numerals in Arabic or Roman numerals:

1. ixss   6. 19

2. XL   7. 39

3. CD   8. $24\frac{1}{4}$

4. LM   9. 240

5. XCIX   10. 499

Concept 3

When converting long Roman numerals to Arabic numerals, it is helpful to separate the Roman numerals into groups and work from both ends.

Example   CDLXXIV → CD L XX IV

      1. Start with the IV = 5 − 1 = 4   4

      2. Next, X+ X = 20   20

      3. C − D = 500 − 100 = 400   400

      4. L = 50   +50

      5. Then add the elements   474

Practice

1. CXIV	6. XLss
2. LVIII	7. CDIV
3. DXIV	8. MCML
4. MDCIXss	9. DXCIIss
5. LXXXIX	10. CMLXXIVss

This method of separating the elements and working from both ends also works well for converting from Arabic to Roman numerals.

Example   Convert 637 to Roman numerals

          600   DC
           30   XXX
            7   VII

    Then rewrite the Roman numeral from the largest number on the left to the smallest numbers on the right. → DCXXXVII

Practice

1. $14\frac{1}{2}$	6. 789
2. 33	7. 450
3. 146	8. 76
4. 329	9. 17
5. 999	10. 1294

Mixed Practice   Convert between Roman numerals and Arabic numerals:

1. DCCL	3. XVIII
2. XXIVss	4. 23

5. 19   13. 362

6. 1,495   14. 16

7. 607   15. 999

8. CCLIVss   16. XXXIXss

9. 66   17. LXXVIII

10. MVII   18. $309\frac{1}{2}$

11. CMVIII   19. 2,515

12. MCDLIV   20. What should you do to convert a number
                                    with decimal 0.5 in it to a Roman numeral?

Time in Allied Health

Universal (military) time is used in many health-care facilities. The Universal time system avoids the confusion over A.M. and P.M. Universal time is based on the 24-hour clock, which begins at 0001, which is one minute after midnight.

Colons are not used between these numbers. Compare the two clocks below:

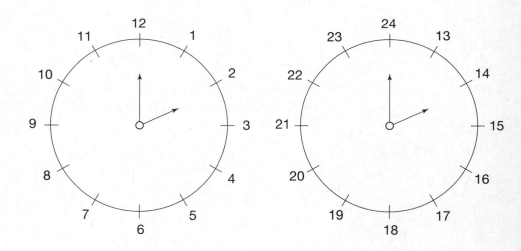

How to Convert to Universal Time:

The hours have four digits: 1 A.M. or 1:00 A.M. = 0100
                                       10 A.M. or 10:00 A.M. = 1000

Add 1200 to any time after noon   2 P.M. or 2:00 P.M. = 1400
                                       2 + 1200 = 1400 in Universal
                                       time
                                       5:36 P.M. or 5:36 P.M. = 1736
                                       in Universal time

Practice 1:   Complete the chart.

Standard Time	Universal or Military Time
12:05 A.M.	_____
3:15 P.M.	_____
7:39 A.M.	_____
7:39 P.M.	_____
12:45 P.M.	_____
8:17 A.M.	_____
5:57 P.M.	_____
1:23 A.M.	_____
9:25 P.M.	_____
11:03 P.M.	_____

Practice 2:   Complete the chart.

Universal or Military Time	Standard Time
1256	_____
0136	_____
0009	_____
1236	_____
0048	_____
2400	_____
1524	_____
2006	_____
0912	_____
1630	_____

WHOLE NUMBER SELF-TEST

1. Complete this number statement. 329 + _____ + 217 = 1,621

2. An activity director in a long-term care facility is purchasing recreational supplies. Find the sum of the purchases: 3 Bingo games at $13

each, 10 puzzles at $9 each, 24 jars of paint at $3 each, and 2 rolls of paper for $31 each.

3. Using the information from problem 2 above, determine the mean (average) cost of these supplies. Round to the nearest dollar.

4. A medical assistant student needs 250 hours of practical work experience to complete the college's course. If the student has completed 184 hours, how many hours remain to fulfill the requirement?

5. Three certified nursing assistants assist 16 rooms of patients on the Saturday morning shift. If each room has 3 patients, how many patients does each assistant care for if they are equally divided up among the staff?

6. Uniform jackets are required at Valley Pharmacy. Each pharmacy technician is asked to purchased two jackets at $21 per jacket and one name badge for $8. What is the cost of these items for each pharmacy technician?

7. The medical clerk is asked to inventory the digital thermometers. In the six examination rooms, the clerk finds the following number of digital thermometers: 2, 4, 5, 2, 1, and 3. The total inventory is _____.

8. The dental assistants in a new office are setting up their free patient sample display. They order the following:

	Quantity	Unit	Item	Per Unit Cost (in dollars)	Total Cost
a.	1,500	each	toothbrush	1	____
b.	100	each	floss (smooth)	2	____
c.	75	each	floss (glide)	2	____
d.	1,000	per 100	information booklet	10	____
e.	25	each	poster	15	____
f.				Subtotal	____

9. After a mild heart attack, Mary spent 3 days in a coronary care unit. Her room bill was $2,898. What was her daily room rate?

10. White blood cell (WBC) count can indicate illness or health. The WBC count of patient B is checked. Before surgery, the WBC count of patient B was 12,674; post-surgery, he had a count of 6,894. What is the difference in patient B's count before and after surgery?

11. The cook has a variety of meals to prepare for Villa Center's residents. She averages 16 vegetarian meals every day of the week. Round the number of weekly meals to the nearest 10.

12. The newest staff member at the hospital is a surgery technologist. Her pay is approximately $14 an hour. If she is scheduled to work 36 hours a week, what is her weekly pay before deductions?

13. Read the number: 956,123.
    The place value of the underlined digit is _____.

Unit 2

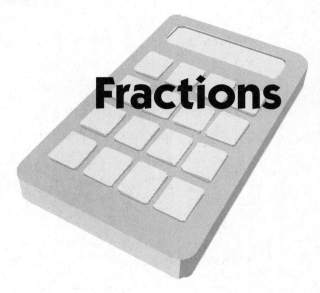

Fractions

Part-to-Whole Relationships

A fraction is a number that has two parts: a part and a whole. A minute is 1 part of 60 minutes in a whole hour. This relationship of part to whole can be shown in a fraction:

$$\frac{1}{60} \begin{array}{l} \leftarrow \text{numerator (the part)} \\ \leftarrow \text{denominator (the whole)} \end{array}$$

The 1 is called the *numerator*, and it represents the part of the whole. The 60 is the *denominator*, and it represents the whole or sum of the parts. Take another common part-to-whole relationship. Many people sleep an average of 8 hours a night. The relationship of sleeping hours to total hours in a day is 8 to 24, or $^8/_{24}$, or a reduced fraction of $^1/_3$.

Fractions are important to know because you will come across them many times in health care occupations. Fractions appear in medication dosages, measurements, sizes of instruments, work assignments, and time units. Practice writing out the numerator (part) to denominator (whole) relationships:

Example

$$\frac{1}{12} = \text{one part to twelve total parts}$$

36

1. $\dfrac{3}{4}$ = _____

2. $\dfrac{5}{6}$ = _____

3. $\dfrac{7}{8}$ = _____

4. $\dfrac{16}{21}$ = _____

Proper or common fractions are fractions with a numerator less than the number of the denominator: $^3/_7$, $^{24}/_{47}$, $^9/_{11}$. The value of any proper or common fraction will be less than 1.

Mixed numbers are fractions that include both a whole number and a proper fraction: $3^3/_4$, $12^9/_{11}$, $101^{13}/_{22}$.

An *improper fraction* has a numerator equal to or larger than the denominator: $^{17}/_{12}$, $^{33}/_{11}$, $^9/_9$. Improper fractions are equal to 1 or larger. Improper fractions are used in the multiplication and division of fractions. Answers that appear as improper fractions need to be reduced so that the answer is a mixed number.

Equivalent Fractions

Understanding *equivalent fractions* is important in making measurement decisions. Equivalent fractions represent the same relationship of part to whole, but there are more pieces or parts involved. The fractions involved, however, are equal. The size of the pieces or parts is what varies.

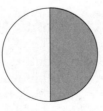   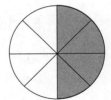

2 large pieces   **8 smaller pieces**
$1/_2$ is shaded   **$4/_8$ are shaded**

The shaded areas are the same size; the number of parts varies. Making fractions equal is easy using multiplication. Look at the fractions: $^1/_6$ and $^?/_{18}$. The denominators are 6 and 18. Ask: 6 times what = 18? The answer is 3, so multiply the numerator by 3, and you will have formed an equivalent fraction. Thus, $^1/_6 = {}^3/_{18}$.

The key to getting the correct answer is in remembering that the number the denominator is multiplied by must also be used to multiply the numerator. If this method is difficult for you, then divide the smaller denominator into the larger one; your answer will then be multiplied by the first numerator to get the second numerator.

$$\frac{1}{6} = \frac{?}{18} \qquad 6\overline{)18,} \qquad \text{then } 3 \times 1 = 3$$

Another way to work this problem is:

$$\frac{1(\times 3)}{6(\times 3)} = \frac{3}{18}$$

Thus, $\frac{1}{6} = \frac{3}{18}$.

Practice

1. $\dfrac{1}{2} = \dfrac{?}{12}$ 6. $\dfrac{1}{13} = \dfrac{?}{39}$

2. $\dfrac{1}{4} = \dfrac{?}{16}$ 7. $\dfrac{4}{8} = \dfrac{?}{72}$

3. $\dfrac{1}{5} = \dfrac{?}{40}$ 8. $\dfrac{1}{5} = \dfrac{?}{100}$

4. $\dfrac{2}{14} = \dfrac{?}{28}$ 9. $\dfrac{7}{9} = \dfrac{42}{?}$

5. $\dfrac{5}{9} = \dfrac{?}{27}$ 10. $\dfrac{1}{3} = \dfrac{8}{?}$

The skill of making equivalent fractions will be used in adding, subtracting, and comparing fractions.

Reducing to Lowest or Simplest Terms

As in making fractions equivalent, reducing fractions to their lowest or simplest terms is another important fraction skill. Most tests and practical applications of fractions require that the answers be in the lowest terms. After each calculation of addition, subtraction, multiplication, or division, you will need to reduce the answer to its lowest terms. Two methods will help you get to the lowest terms:

Multiplication Method

To use the multiplication method, look at the numbers in the fraction. Find a number that divides into both the numerator and denominator evenly. Such numbers are called *factors* of the numbers. Write out the multiplication for the numerator and denominator. Cross out the two identical numbers in the multiplication problems. What is left will be the reduced fraction.

$$\frac{2}{16} = \frac{2 \times 1}{2 \times 8} \rightarrow \frac{\cancel{2} \times 1}{\cancel{2} \times 8}$$

So, $^2/_6 = ^1/_8$. Depending on the multiple you choose, you may need to do this more than once.

$$\frac{8}{24} = \frac{4 \times 2}{4 \times 6} = \frac{2}{6} \rightarrow \frac{1}{3}$$

or

$$\frac{8}{24} = \frac{8 \times 1}{8 \times 3} = \frac{1}{3}$$

Sometimes students only partially reduce a fraction, so try to find the largest possible factor of the numbers when you are reducing.

> Choose the largest possible multiple to avoid having to repeat the steps in reduction.

Division Method

Look at the numbers of the numerator and the denominator. Choose a number that divides into both the numerator and the denominator. Next, divide the numerator and denominator by that number. Check to ensure that the resulting fraction is in its lowest form.

$$\frac{2}{16} = \frac{2 \div 2}{16 \div 2} = \frac{1}{8}$$

$$\frac{8}{24} = \frac{8 \div 4}{24 \div 4} = \frac{2}{6}$$

This fraction is not reduced, so it must be reduced again.

$$\frac{2}{6} = \frac{2 \div 2}{6 \div 2} = \frac{1}{3}$$

This fraction is reduced to its lowest form.

How do you decide on the best method to use?

Choose your strongest skill—multiplication or division—and use it to reduce fractions.

You will make fewer errors if you select one method and use it consistently.

Practice   1. $\dfrac{2}{14}$ 4. $\dfrac{13}{39}$

2. $\dfrac{3}{27}$ 5. $\dfrac{25}{100}$

3. $\dfrac{4}{8}$ 6. $\dfrac{64}{72}$

7. $\dfrac{24}{48}$ 9. $\dfrac{15}{45}$

8. $\dfrac{63}{90}$ 10. $\dfrac{5}{255}$

When working with a mixed number, set aside the whole number. Handle the fraction portion of the number and then place it beside the whole number.

$$14\dfrac{3}{9} \rightarrow 14 \text{ and } \dfrac{3}{9} \rightarrow \dfrac{3}{9} = \dfrac{1 \times 3}{3 \times 3} = \dfrac{1}{3} \rightarrow 14\dfrac{1}{3}$$

> Set aside the whole number, reduce the fraction, then replace the whole number next to the reduced fraction.

Practice   1. $13\dfrac{2}{8}$

2. $7\dfrac{12}{16}$

3. $1\dfrac{33}{66}$

4. $2\dfrac{2}{20}$

5. $3\dfrac{3}{12}$

6. $5\dfrac{14}{64}$

7. $2\dfrac{11}{99}$

8. $10\dfrac{30}{80}$

9. $6\dfrac{45}{90}$

10. $4\dfrac{22}{30}$

Fractional parts or relationships are common in health care.

Example   In a class of 30 people, 13 students are male and 17 are female. To write the relationship of the number of males to the total number of students, we place the part (13) over the whole (30) or total number of students.

$$\dfrac{13}{30}$$

Practice   Write th...
whole. The...

1. 50 of the 125...

2. The dietitian uses...
   breakfast. Represent...
   to eight-ounce glasses u...

3. 30 out of 90 patients at the s...
   the fractional part of women to...

4. 14 female babies and 16 male babies...
   female babies to male babies as a fractio...

5. About 500 medicine cups are used daily at a...
   nurse claims that approximately 4,000 medicin...
   What is the day-to-week use rate of medicine cups...

Improper Fractions

Working with improper fractions also requires reducing fract...
improper fraction is a fraction that has a larger numerator...
denominator.

$$\frac{16}{8} = \frac{8 \times 2 = 2}{8 \times 1 = 1} \rightarrow 2$$

If the numerator and the denominator do not have a common number by which the numbers can be multiplied, simply divide the denominator into the numerator.

$$\frac{11}{8} \qquad 8\overline{)11} \; 1\frac{3}{8}$$
$$\frac{8}{3}$$

The remainder 3 is a whole number. Place it on top of the divisor to form a fraction.

Improper fractions are either whole numbers or mixed numbers.
Improper fractions are used for dividing mixed numbers.

Practice

1. $\dfrac{15}{2}$

2. $\dfrac{18}{4}$

3. $\dfrac{39}{2}$

fractional part that represents the relationships of the part to the
reduce all your answers to the lowest form.

patients see the physical therapist each week.

35 six-ounce glasses and 50 eight-ounce glasses at
in fraction form the relationship of six-ounce glasses
used at breakfast.

hort-term care facility are women. What is
total patients?

were born on Saturday. Express the

long-term care facility. The
cups are used a week.

ions. An
han a

forward. Follow

s, and place the

ccuracy.

$$+\frac{5}{6} \qquad +\frac{9}{8} \qquad \text{Reduce by } 9 \div 8 = 1\frac{1}{8}$$

When reducing the answer, you find that the result is a whole number with a 1 for its denominator. In this case, use the numerator, a whole number alone. Do not use the 1 since the answer is actually a whole number rather than a fraction.

Step 1:
$$\frac{12}{15} \\ +\frac{18}{15} \\ \hline \frac{30}{15}$$

Step 2: $\dfrac{30}{15} = \dfrac{\cancel{15} \times 2}{\cancel{15} \times 1} \qquad \dfrac{2}{1} = 2$

If a whole number exists with the fractions, simply add it separately and place the fraction next to the answer. The whole number will be affected only if the fraction answer is larger than 1—then the whole number resulting from the fraction addition is added to the whole number answer.

Example

$$14\frac{2}{8}$$
$$+7\frac{1}{8}$$
$$\overline{21\frac{3}{8}}$$

Add the fractions: $\frac{2}{8} + \frac{1}{8} = \frac{3}{8}$

Add the whole numbers: $14 + 7 = 21$

Write the answer. No reduction is necessary.

Example

$$10\frac{2}{4}$$
$$+4\frac{3}{4}$$
$$\overline{14\frac{5}{4}}$$

Add the fractions: $\frac{2}{4} + \frac{3}{4} = \frac{5}{4}$

Add $10 + 4 = 14$

$\frac{5}{4}$ must be reduced. It is an improper fraction.

Divide 5 by $4 = 1\frac{1}{4}$. The whole number 1 is added to 14 $(14 + 1 = 15)$ and the fraction $\frac{1}{4}$ is placed next to the whole so that the answer is $15\frac{1}{4}$.

Practice Add the following fractions. Reduce as necessary:

1. $\frac{1}{6} + \frac{5}{6}$

2. $\frac{2}{8} + \frac{4}{8}$

3. $\frac{9}{10} + \frac{11}{10}$

4. $\frac{1}{13} + \frac{4}{13}$

5. $\frac{3}{12} + \frac{4}{12}$

6. $\frac{2}{5} + \frac{3}{5}$

7. $\frac{3}{13} + \frac{4}{13}$

8. $13\frac{8}{12} + 2\frac{2}{12}$

9. $10\frac{1}{6} + 12\frac{4}{6}$

10. $11\frac{1}{4} + \frac{3}{4}$

11. $\frac{3}{5} + \frac{1}{5}$

12. $\frac{2}{7} + \frac{3}{7} + \frac{4}{7}$

13. $\frac{3}{8} + \frac{4}{8} + \frac{1}{8}$

14. $2\frac{1}{12} + 3\frac{5}{12} + 6\frac{4}{12}$

15. $101\frac{3}{4} + 33\frac{1}{4} + 5\frac{1}{4}$

Finding the Common Denominator

Adding and subtracting fractions requires that the denominator be of the same number, also referred to as a *common denominator*. The lowest common denominator is the smallest number or multiple that both of the denominators of the fractions can go into.

By using multiplication, find a smallest number or multiple that the numbers can go into.

Step 1:

$$\frac{2}{3} \quad \underline{\quad\quad} \quad = ?$$
$$3 \times 2 = 6$$
$$+\frac{1}{6} \rightarrow \quad\quad \frac{1}{6}$$

In the above problem, 3 and 6 are the denominators. $3 \times 2 = 6$, so 6 is the common denominator.

Step 2: Once you have the common denominator in place, multiply the numerator by the same number with which you multiplied the denominator. The result will be equivalent fractions, so the number relationships remain the same.

$$\frac{2}{3} \quad \frac{2 \times 2 = 4}{3 \times 2 = 6}$$
$$+\frac{1}{6} \rightarrow \quad +\frac{1}{6}$$
$$\frac{5}{6}$$

Practice   Find the common denominator in the following pairs of numbers. Set the problems up vertically and think about their multiples to find the common denominators.

> Fewer errors occur if the setup is vertical. You can see the numbers and their relationships easier.

1. $\frac{2}{4}$ and $\frac{1}{5}$

2. $\frac{3}{8}$ and $\frac{1}{16}$

3. $\frac{22}{44}$ and $\frac{1}{11}$

4. $\frac{1}{9}$ and $\frac{5}{45}$

5. $\frac{2}{5}$ and $\frac{3}{25}$

6. $\frac{3}{7}$ and $\frac{9}{49}$

7. $\frac{1}{200}$ and $\frac{5}{20}$

8. $\frac{4}{50}$ and $\frac{10}{150}$

9. $\frac{3}{9}$ and $\frac{4}{27}$

10. $\frac{1}{6}$ and $\frac{4}{18}$

Practice Add the following fractions with unlike denominators:

1. $\frac{3}{5} + \frac{1}{4}$

2. $\frac{1}{2} + \frac{4}{6}$

3. $\frac{4}{9} + \frac{2}{3}$

4. $\frac{7}{10} + \frac{3}{5}$

5. $\frac{11}{30} + \frac{2}{15}$

6. $\frac{5}{25} + \frac{1}{5}$

7. $\frac{4}{7} + \frac{1}{21}$

8. $\frac{2}{5} + \frac{1}{10} + \frac{3}{10}$

9. $\frac{3}{5} + \frac{1}{3} + \frac{2}{15}$

10. $\frac{2}{3} + \frac{1}{12} + \frac{2}{4}$

11. $\dfrac{1}{10} + \dfrac{1}{2} + \dfrac{4}{5}$

12. $12\dfrac{1}{6} + \dfrac{3}{4}$

13. $55\dfrac{1}{3} + 51\dfrac{5}{9}$

14. $5\dfrac{1}{2} + 2\dfrac{4}{5} + 5\dfrac{3}{10}$

15. $4\dfrac{3}{4} + 1\dfrac{1}{16} + 3\dfrac{2}{32}$

Sometimes one must consider a wider range of possible numbers for common denominators. For example, you may have a pair of fractions in which one of the denominators cannot be multiplied by a number to get the other denominator. In this case, it is often easiest to simply multiply the two denominators with each other. The result will be a common denominator.

Example

$$\dfrac{3}{13} \text{ and } \dfrac{1}{4}$$

What is the common denominator? If you multiply 13×4, your answer is 52. Use that number as the common denominator.

> To find the more difficult common denominators, multiply the denominators with each other.

$$\dfrac{3}{13} \rightarrow 13 \times 4 = 52$$

$$\dfrac{1}{4} \rightarrow 4 \times 13 = 52$$

Then multiply each numerator by the same number that you multiplied its denominator by. Do this for each fraction and the result will be a common denominator.

$$\dfrac{3}{13} \rightarrow \dfrac{3 \times 4 = 12}{13 \times 4 = 52}$$

$$\dfrac{1}{4} \rightarrow \dfrac{1 \times 13 = 13}{4 \times 13 = 52}$$

By finding the common denominator, you have also created equivalent fractions.

Practice Find the common denominator for each of the following sets of fractions:

1. $\dfrac{3}{4}$ and $\dfrac{2}{5}$

2. $\dfrac{7}{8}$ and $\dfrac{1}{3}$

3. $\dfrac{24}{32}$ and $\dfrac{1}{6}$

4. $\dfrac{1}{7}$ and $\dfrac{4}{8}$

5. $\dfrac{3}{5}$ and $\dfrac{7}{9}$

6. $\dfrac{2}{26}$ and $\dfrac{1}{3}$

7. $\dfrac{3}{9}$ and $\dfrac{1}{4}$

8. $\dfrac{2}{5}$ and $\dfrac{6}{9}$

9. $\dfrac{3}{10}$ and $\dfrac{2}{3}$

10. $\dfrac{1}{9}$ and $\dfrac{7}{8}$

Practice Add the following mixed fractions:

1. $3\dfrac{2}{3} + 6\dfrac{1}{4}$

2. $10\dfrac{1}{2} + 13\dfrac{5}{22}$

3. $9\dfrac{1}{6} + 4\dfrac{3}{9}$

4. $11\dfrac{7}{8} + 2\dfrac{1}{7}$

5. $\dfrac{1}{2} + 4\dfrac{1}{7} + 2\dfrac{1}{14}$

6. $12\dfrac{3}{5} + 22\dfrac{1}{30}$

7. $10\dfrac{4}{5} + 8\dfrac{1}{6}$

8. $3\dfrac{4}{9} + 1\dfrac{2}{3} + 5\dfrac{2}{9}$

9. $11\dfrac{2}{5} + 7\dfrac{1}{2}$

10. $7\dfrac{11}{16} + 3\dfrac{4}{8} + \dfrac{1}{2}$

11. $2\dfrac{2}{9} + 6\dfrac{1}{3} + 8\dfrac{2}{27}$

12. $6\dfrac{2}{3} + 8\dfrac{4}{5} + 3\dfrac{6}{10}$

13. $6\dfrac{1}{4} + 13\dfrac{2}{3} + 19\dfrac{1}{2}$

14. $6\dfrac{7}{16} + \dfrac{3}{24} + 2\dfrac{1}{48}$

15. $\dfrac{3}{5} + \dfrac{6}{30} + 12\dfrac{2}{3}$

16. $8\dfrac{9}{11} + 3\dfrac{1}{33} + \dfrac{2}{66}$

17. $3\dfrac{5}{16} + \dfrac{5}{8} + \dfrac{2}{4}$

18. $\dfrac{5}{6} + 3\dfrac{3}{9} + 7\dfrac{2}{3}$

19. $4\dfrac{5}{6} + \dfrac{2}{5} + \dfrac{4}{15}$

20. $55\dfrac{4}{17} + 101\dfrac{3}{51}$

Applications

1. The certified nurse assistants weigh patients each month. Mrs. Smith weighed 120 pounds last month. Over the last two months, she gained $1\frac{1}{2}$ and $\frac{1}{4}$ pounds. What is Mrs. Smith's current weight?

2. The lab technician uses a cleaning solution daily. The technician used $4\frac{1}{2}$ ounces, $1\frac{1}{3}$ ounces, and 5 ounces of the cleaning solutions. What is the total amount of solution used?

3. A new baby grew $\frac{3}{4}$ of an inch in June and $\frac{7}{16}$ of an inch in July. How many total inches did the baby grow during these two months?

4. A sick child drinks $\frac{1}{2}$ cup of juice and an hour later $\frac{3}{4}$ cup of water. At dinner, the child drinks $1\frac{1}{4}$ cups more of water. What is the child's total fluid intake?

5. The nurse gives a patient $1\frac{1}{2}$ grains of medication followed by $2\frac{1}{3}$ grains. What is the total dosage the nurse has dispensed to the patient?

Ordering Fractions

Comparing fractions in health-care fields appears when sizes of medical items or pieces of equipment are being computed. It is useful to be able to determine the size relationships of instruments and place them in order for a surgeon before a surgery. This is accomplished by using the common denominator method.

Know these symbols: $<, =, >$

3 is less than 4 is represented by $3 < 4$

7 is greater than 5 is represented by $7 > 5$

$\frac{2}{2}$ equals 1 is represented by $\frac{2}{2} = 1$

Example Which is larger $\frac{1}{4}$ or $\frac{3}{8}$?

Step 1: Convert the fractions to give each a common denominator.

$$\frac{1}{4} \qquad \begin{array}{l} 1 \times 2 = 2 \\ 4 \times 2 = 8 \end{array}$$

$$\frac{3}{8} \rightarrow \qquad \frac{3}{8}$$

Step 2: Order by the numerators now that the fractions have the same denominator. 3 is larger than 2, so $\frac{3}{8} > \frac{2}{8}$ or $\frac{1}{4}$.

Practice Order the following fractions from largest to smallest.

1. $\dfrac{1}{4}, \dfrac{2}{9}, \dfrac{4}{12}$

2. $\dfrac{9}{22}, \dfrac{5}{11}, \dfrac{8}{11}$

3. $\dfrac{6}{25}, \dfrac{20}{50}, \dfrac{33}{100}$

4. $\dfrac{7}{8}, \dfrac{2}{16}, \dfrac{3}{4}, \dfrac{1}{2}$

Subtraction of Fractions

Subtraction of fractions follows the same basic principles as addition of fractions. The fractions must have common denominators before any subtraction can be done.

Example **Step 1:** Make a common denominator if necessary.

$$\frac{7}{8} - \frac{5}{8} = \underline{\quad} \text{ (8 is the common denominator.)}$$

Step 2: Subtract the numerators and then reduce if necessary.

$$\frac{7}{8} - \frac{5}{8} = \frac{2}{8}, \text{ which is reduced to } \frac{1}{4}.$$

Practice

1. $\dfrac{3}{9} - \dfrac{2}{9}$

2. $\dfrac{5}{8} - \dfrac{2}{8}$

3. $\dfrac{3}{11} - \dfrac{1}{11}$

4. $\dfrac{22}{44} - \dfrac{11}{44}$

5. $10\dfrac{5}{12} - 8\dfrac{3}{12}$

6. $25\dfrac{3}{4} - 20\dfrac{1}{4}$

7. $101\dfrac{13}{24} - 56\dfrac{10}{24}$

8. $6\dfrac{6}{7} - \dfrac{3}{5}$

9. $\dfrac{15}{16} - \dfrac{7}{16}$

10. $20\dfrac{5}{6} - 12\dfrac{2}{6}$

11. $\dfrac{3}{4} - \dfrac{1}{2}$

12. $\dfrac{6}{8} - \dfrac{1}{4}$

13. $12\dfrac{1}{2} - \dfrac{3}{10}$

14. $20\dfrac{6}{14} - 2\dfrac{3}{7}$

15. $39\dfrac{11}{18} - 8\dfrac{3}{6}$

16. $25\dfrac{1}{3} - 20\dfrac{1}{8}$

17. $124\dfrac{11}{12} - \dfrac{5}{6}$

18. $18\dfrac{3}{4} - 12\dfrac{2}{3}$

19. $200\dfrac{9}{11} - 188\dfrac{2}{3}$

20. $500\dfrac{4}{5} - 150\dfrac{2}{9}$

Borrowing in Subtraction of Fractions

Two specific situations require that a number be borrowed in the subtraction of fractions: (1) subtraction of a fraction from a whole number, and (2) after a common denominator is established and the top fraction of the problem is less or smaller than the fraction that is being subtracted from it.

Recall that the borrowing in whole numbers is accomplished as shown below. Set the problem up vertically.

$$124 - 8 = \underline{\hspace{1cm}}$$

Step 1: Borrow 1 from the tens column. Add it to the ones column.

Step 2: Subtract.

$$1^1 2^1 4$$
$$\underline{-8}$$
$$116$$

In fractions, the same borrowing concept is used; the format varies only slightly. The difference is that the borrowed number must be put into a fractional form.

> Any whole number over itself equals 1. So $^{101}/_{101} = 1$, $^3/_3 = 1$, and $^{12}/_{12} = 1$.

Example

$$17\frac{3}{8}$$
$$-14\frac{4}{8}$$

In the example above, the numerator 4 in the second fraction cannot be subtracted from the first fraction's numerator 3. Thus, borrowing is required in the first fraction.

$$1^6 \not{7}\frac{3}{8} + \frac{8}{8}$$
$$-14\frac{4}{8}$$

Step 1: Borrow 1 from the whole number. Convert the 1 into an improper fraction having the same common denominator as the first fraction. Then add the two fractions.

Step 2: Rewrite the problem so it incorporates the changes, then subtract the numerator only. Place it over the denominator. Reduce as necessary.

$$16\frac{11}{8}$$
$$-14\frac{4}{8}$$
$$2\frac{7}{8}$$

Borrowing in Subtraction Rules

1. Must have a common denominator.
2. To borrow from the whole number, make it a fractional part.
3. Add fractional parts.
4. Subtract; reduce if necessary.

Practice

1. $11 - \dfrac{5}{6}$

2. $9 - \dfrac{3}{5}$

3. $10 - \dfrac{2}{8}$

4. $13 - \dfrac{5}{9}$

5. $15 - \dfrac{7}{13}$

6. $30 - \dfrac{4}{11}$

7. $8\dfrac{2}{7} - 2\dfrac{3}{7}$

8. $14\dfrac{3}{12} - 10\dfrac{10}{12}$

9. $15\dfrac{1}{5} - 4\dfrac{4}{5}$

10. $9\dfrac{2}{4} - 5\dfrac{3}{4}$

Remember that when you are subtracting, the first rule is that you must have a common denominator. Once the common denominator is in place, borrow if necessary. Then subtract, placing the answer over the denominator; reduce as necessary.

Practice

1. $14\dfrac{2}{5} - 6\dfrac{3}{4}$

2. $34\dfrac{1}{4} - 10\dfrac{4}{5}$

3. $36\dfrac{1}{6} - 16\dfrac{3}{5}$

4. $13\dfrac{3}{4} - 7\dfrac{7}{8}$

5. $16\frac{3}{11} - 10\frac{1}{2}$

6. $19\frac{1}{2} - 15\frac{7}{12}$

7. $112\frac{1}{2} - \frac{11}{15}$

8. $18\frac{3}{7} - 2\frac{7}{14}$

9. $45\frac{3}{8} - 13\frac{3}{4}$

10. $125\frac{2}{12} - 28\frac{5}{6}$

11. $29\frac{1}{4} - 12\frac{5}{12}$

12. $12\frac{1}{6} - 1\frac{4}{5}$

13. $90\frac{4}{9} - 13\frac{3}{4}$

14. $28\frac{1}{7} - 4\frac{6}{7}$

15. $13\frac{2}{20} - 6\frac{6}{10}$

Additional Practice

1. $12\frac{1}{2} - 4\frac{7}{8}$

2. $14 - \frac{3}{7}$

3. $12\frac{1}{16} - 2\frac{5}{16}$

4. $20\frac{2}{3} - 10\frac{7}{9}$

5. $54\frac{1}{2} - 42\frac{3}{4}$

6. $22\frac{3}{5} - 17\frac{5}{6}$

7. $87 - 14\frac{2}{7}$

8. $225\frac{1}{4} - 34\frac{3}{8}$

9. $90\dfrac{1}{3} - 6\dfrac{3}{4}$

10. $45 - \dfrac{15}{16}$

Application

1. A patient is on a low sodium, low fat diet. Three months ago the patient weighed $210\frac{1}{4}$ pounds. Now the patient weighs $198\frac{3}{4}$ pounds. How many pounds did the patient lose?

2. The school nurse encourages all students to drink at least 4 pints of water daily. Most students drink at least $1\frac{1}{2}$ pints. How much additional water should the students consume?

3. The pharmacy technician helps with annual inventory. If there were 125 boxes of computer labels at the beginning of the inventory period, and $25\frac{3}{4}$ remain, how many boxes of labels were used throughout the year?

4. The dietitian had a 100 pound bag of unbleached flour at the beginning of the month. If she used $73\frac{1}{2}$ pounds, how much flour does she have left?

5. The recreation center is helping residents make placemats for the holidays. Each resident is given 45 inches of decorative edging per placemat. If each placemat uses $41\frac{1}{2}$ inches of decorative edging, how much edging is left over from each placemat?

Multiplication of Fractions

To facilitate multiplication and division of fractions, set up the problems horizontally.

One of the simplest computations in fractions is to multiply a common fraction. No common denominator is needed.

Example

Step 1: Set up the problem horizontally and multiply the fraction straight across.

$$\dfrac{7 \times 1 \rightarrow}{8 \times 4 \rightarrow} = \dfrac{7}{32}$$

Step 2: Reduce to the lowest terms, if necessary. $\frac{7}{32}$ does not need to be reduced.

Practice

1. $\dfrac{3}{4} \times \dfrac{1}{12}$

2. $\dfrac{1}{2} \times \dfrac{4}{5}$

3. $\dfrac{7}{9} \times \dfrac{4}{5}$

4. $\dfrac{2}{3} \times \dfrac{4}{6}$

5. $\dfrac{1}{5} \times \dfrac{3}{7}$

6. $\dfrac{12}{48} \times \dfrac{1}{2}$

7. $\dfrac{6}{9} \times \dfrac{2}{3}$

8. $\dfrac{10}{100} \times \dfrac{2}{5}$

9. $\dfrac{1}{3} \times \dfrac{13}{22}$

10. $\dfrac{4}{5} \times \dfrac{1}{20}$

Review some number concepts in fractions that will help ensure accurate answers.

> Any number over itself equals 1: $\frac{4}{4}$, $\frac{8}{8}$, and $\frac{105}{105}$ all equal 1.
> Any numerator that has 1 as its denominator should be represented as a whole number:
>
> $$\frac{4}{1} = 4, \ \frac{6}{1} = 6, \ \frac{51}{1} = 51, \text{ and } \frac{102}{1} = 102$$

Multiplying a Fraction by a Whole Number

To multiply a fraction by a whole number, follow these steps:

Example

$$\frac{1}{6} \times 2 = \underline{\qquad}$$

Step 1: Make the whole number into a fraction by placing a 1 as its denominator.

$$\frac{1}{6} \times \frac{2}{1}$$

> Any whole number can become a fraction by placing a 1 as the denominator. $14 = {}^{14}/_1$

Step 2: Multiply straight across and then reduce if necessary.

$$\frac{1}{6} \times \frac{2}{1} = \frac{2}{6} \rightarrow \frac{1}{3}$$

Reduce to $\frac{1}{3}$.

Practice

1. $\frac{1}{4} \times 6$

2. $3 \times \frac{2}{5}$

3. $\frac{7}{15} \times 35$

4. $24 \times \frac{2}{7}$

5. $7 \times \frac{8}{10}$

6. $16 \times \frac{1}{3}$

7. $\frac{5}{9} \times 21$

8. $\frac{5}{30} \times 200$

9. $\frac{1}{8} \times 32$

10. $\frac{11}{50} \times 20$

Reducing before You Multiply as a Timesaver

When multiplying, you can expedite the work by reducing before you multiply. This is useful because it relies on the multiples of the numbers to reduce the numbers you are multiplying. This saves time at the end of the problem because you won't have to spend so much time reducing the answer.

Look at the numbers involved in $^2/_5 \times {}^3/_4$. If a numerator number can go into a denominator number evenly, then canceling is possible.

$$\frac{{}^1 2}{5} \times \frac{3}{4_2} \qquad \text{The 2 goes into the 4 twice because } 2 \times 2 = 4$$

Then multiply the changed numerals straight across.

$$\frac{1 \times 3}{5 \times 2} = \frac{3}{10}$$

The answer is $^3/_{10}$. If the problem was done without canceling, the answer after multiplication would be $^6/_{20}$, which needs to be reduced to $^3/_{10}$. Reducing first saves time by allowing you to work with smaller numbers. For more complicated problems, it may be easier to cancel by writing out the number involved.

Example   **Step 1:** Write out the multiples of each number to find numbers that each can go into evenly.

$$(10 \times 1) \qquad (3 \times 1)$$
$$\frac{10}{15} \qquad \times \qquad \frac{3}{100}$$
$$(3 \times 5) \qquad (10 \times 10)$$

Step 2: Then, begin by crossing out the matching numbers, working from top to bottom and crossing out like numbers. Cross out the matching numbers.

$$(\cancel{10} \times 1) \qquad (\cancel{3} \times 1)$$
$$\frac{10}{15} \qquad \times \qquad \frac{3}{100}$$
$$(\cancel{3} \times 5) \qquad (\cancel{10} \times 10)$$

Step 3: Then multiply the remaining numbers straight across.

$$
\left.
\begin{array}{l}
(\cancel{10} \times 1) \quad (\cancel{3} \times 1) \quad \to 1 \times 1 = \underline{1} \\[4pt]
\dfrac{10}{15} \quad \times \quad \dfrac{3}{100} \\[4pt]
(\cancel{3} \times 5) \quad (\cancel{10} \times 10) \quad \to 5 \times 10 = 50
\end{array}
\right\} \dfrac{1}{50}
$$

When there are more than two fractions, reducing of fractions can occur anywhere within the fraction as long as the reducing is done by the top and bottom numbers. There can be multiple reductions of fractions as well.
   For example:

$$\frac{11}{16} \times \frac{3}{12} \times \frac{8}{66} \to \quad \text{Set the problem up using the factors for each number.}$$

$$(11 \times 1) \quad (3 \times 1) \quad (2 \times 4)$$
$$\frac{11}{16} \qquad \times \qquad \frac{3}{12} \qquad \times \qquad \frac{8}{66}$$
$$(2 \times 8) \quad (4 \times 3) \quad (6 \times 11)$$

$$\left.\begin{array}{ccc}
(\cancel{11} \times 1) & (\cancel{3} \times 1) & (\cancel{2} \times 4) \\
\dfrac{11}{16} \times & \dfrac{3}{12} \times & \dfrac{8}{66} \\
(\cancel{2} \times 8) & (4 \times \cancel{3}) & (6 \times \cancel{11})
\end{array}\right\} \quad \text{After reducing, multiply to get } \dfrac{1}{48}$$

Practice

1. $\dfrac{4}{5} \times \dfrac{15}{7}$

2. $\dfrac{12}{20} \times \dfrac{4}{24}$

3. $\dfrac{3}{7} \times \dfrac{21}{36}$

4. $\dfrac{5}{6} \times \dfrac{3}{30}$

5. $\dfrac{11}{15} \times \dfrac{3}{44}$

6. $\dfrac{3}{7} \times \dfrac{7}{11}$

7. $\dfrac{14}{20} \times \dfrac{10}{28}$

8. $\dfrac{1}{3} \times \dfrac{3}{6} \times \dfrac{2}{4}$

9. $\dfrac{11}{16} \times \dfrac{4}{12} \times \dfrac{22}{44}$

10. $\dfrac{9}{10} \times \dfrac{1}{3} \times \dfrac{8}{13}$

11. $\dfrac{8}{14} \times \dfrac{25}{48} \times \dfrac{7}{50}$

12. $\dfrac{5}{12} \times \dfrac{33}{34} \times \dfrac{17}{20} \times \dfrac{60}{66}$

Multiplication of Mixed Numbers

Mixed numbers are whole numbers with fractions. Multiplication involving mixed numbers requires that the mixed number be changed to an improper fraction.

Example Change $1\frac{3}{4}$ into an improper fraction.

Step 1: Multiply the whole number times the denominator, then add the numerator.

$$1\frac{3}{4} \rightarrow 1 \times 4 + 3 = 7$$

Step 2: Place the answer from step 1 over the denominator.

$$1\frac{3}{4} \rightarrow \quad 1 \times 4 + 3 = 7 \quad \rightarrow \quad \frac{7}{4}$$

$$\frac{7}{4} \quad \text{So } 1\frac{3}{4} = \frac{7}{4}$$

This improper fraction is not further reduced or changed. It may now be multiplied by another fraction.

Practice   Change these mixed numbers into improper fractions.

1. $8\frac{1}{4}$

2. $5\frac{2}{3}$

3. $17\frac{3}{5}$

4. $24\frac{4}{7}$

5. $2\frac{3}{12}$

6. $4\frac{3}{8}$

7. $3\frac{5}{9}$

8. $12\frac{1}{4}$

9. $4\frac{5}{12}$

10. $10\frac{1}{3}$

After converting mixed numbers to improper fractions, continue by following the same rules as for multiplying common fractions.

Example $\frac{1}{3} \times 5\frac{1}{4}$

Step 1: Change the mixed number into an improper fraction.

$$5\frac{1}{4} \rightarrow 5 \times 4 = 20 + 1 = \frac{21}{4}$$

Step 2: Reduce, if possible.

$$\frac{1}{3} \times \frac{\overset{(3 \times 7)}{21}}{\underset{(3 \times 1)}{4}}$$

Step 3: Multiply straight across.

$$\begin{array}{l} 1 \times 7 = 7 \\ \overline{1 \times 4 = 4} \end{array}$$

Step 4: Change the improper fraction to a mixed fraction.

$$\frac{7}{4} \rightarrow 7 \div 4 = 1\frac{3}{4}$$

Example

$$3\frac{1}{4} \times 5\frac{2}{5}$$

Step 1: Change to improper fractions.

$$3\frac{1}{4} \rightarrow 3 \times 4 = 12 + 1 = \frac{13}{4} \quad \text{and}$$

$$5\frac{2}{5} \rightarrow 5 \times 5 = 25 + 2 = \frac{27}{5}$$

Step 2: Reduce, if possible.

$$\frac{13}{4} \times \frac{27}{5} \text{ — not possible}$$

Step 3: Multiply straight across.

$$\frac{13}{4} \times \frac{27}{5} = \frac{351}{20}$$

Step 4: Reduce — Divide 351 by 20. Write it as a mixed fraction.

$$\begin{array}{r} 17\frac{11}{20} \\ 20\overline{)351} \\ 20\downarrow \\ \overline{151} \\ 140 \\ \overline{11} \end{array} \qquad \text{Answer: } 17\frac{11}{20}$$

Practice

1. $2\dfrac{5}{12} \times \dfrac{1}{7}$

2. $4\dfrac{2}{3} \times \dfrac{4}{5}$

3. $\dfrac{3}{10} \times 1\dfrac{3}{4}$

4. $2\dfrac{1}{8} \times \dfrac{6}{11}$

5. $\dfrac{4}{9} \times 1\dfrac{2}{3}$

6. $3\dfrac{5}{7} \times 2\dfrac{5}{14}$

7. $17\dfrac{1}{4} \times 2\dfrac{1}{3}$

8. $1\dfrac{1}{4} \times 2\dfrac{1}{5}$

9. $2\dfrac{1}{5} \times 1\dfrac{3}{4}$

10. $3\dfrac{1}{6} \times 3\dfrac{1}{4}$

Applications

1. A bottle of medicine contains 30 doses. How many doses are in $2\frac{1}{3}$ bottles?

2. The nurse worked a total of $2\frac{1}{4}$ hours overtime. She is paid $32 an hour for overtime work. What are her overtime earnings?

3. One tablet contains 250 milligrams of pain medication. How many milligrams are in $3\frac{1}{2}$ tablets?

4. One cup holds 8 ounces of liquid. If a cup is $\frac{2}{3}$ full, how many ounces are in the cup?

5. The dietitian is working in a long-term care residence. Each day she prepares a high protein drink for 25 residents. If each drink measures $\frac{3}{4}$ cup, how many total cups of the drink will she prepare a day?

Division of Fractions

To divide fractions, two steps are required to compute the answer.

Example Solve: $\dfrac{1}{8} \div \dfrac{1}{4} =$ _____

Step 1: Change the sign to a × sign.

$$\frac{1}{8} \div \frac{1}{4} \rightarrow \frac{1}{8} \times \frac{1}{4}$$

Step 2: Invert the fraction to the right of the ÷ sign.

$$\frac{1}{8} \div \frac{1}{4} \rightarrow \frac{1}{8} \times \frac{4}{1}$$

This inversion causes the fraction to change from $\frac{1}{4}$ to $\frac{4}{1}$, which is called the reciprocal of $\frac{1}{4}$.

> The reciprocal of any fraction is its inverse:
>
> $$\frac{2}{3} \rightarrow \frac{3}{2} \qquad \frac{12}{35} \rightarrow \frac{35}{12} \quad \text{and} \quad \frac{9}{11} \rightarrow \frac{11}{9}$$

Step 3: Follow the steps of multiplication of fractions: Reduce if possible; then multiply straight across and reduce as necessary.

$$
\begin{array}{c}
(4 \times 1) \\
\text{Reduce} \quad \frac{1}{8} \times \frac{4}{1} = \quad \frac{1}{2} \\
(4 \times 2)
\end{array}
$$

Example Solve: $\dfrac{4}{9} \div \dfrac{1}{3} =$ _____

Step 1: Change the ÷ sign to an × sign.

$$\frac{4}{9} \times \frac{1}{3}$$

Step 2: Invert the fraction after the ÷ sign.

$$\frac{4}{9} \times \frac{3}{1}$$

Step 3: Multiply straight across.

$$\frac{4}{9} \times \frac{3}{1} = \frac{12}{9} \qquad \begin{array}{r} 1\frac{3}{9} \\ 9\overline{)12} \\ \underline{-9} \end{array}$$

Reduce

The answer is $1\frac{3}{9}$. Note $\frac{3}{9}$ reduces to $\frac{1}{3}$, so the answer is $1\frac{1}{3}$.

Practice

1. $\dfrac{3}{7} \div \dfrac{3}{5}$

2. $\dfrac{5}{35} \div \dfrac{11}{21}$

3. $\dfrac{3}{12} \div \dfrac{6}{7}$

4. $\dfrac{7}{9} \div \dfrac{4}{5}$

5. $\dfrac{8}{9} \div \dfrac{1}{9}$

6. $33 \div \dfrac{11}{12}$

7. $\dfrac{1}{3} \div 15$

8. $6 \div \dfrac{1}{3}$

9. $\dfrac{7}{28} \div 30$

10. $8\dfrac{6}{10} \div 1\dfrac{4}{5}$

11. $4\dfrac{3}{8} \div 1\dfrac{2}{16}$

12. $7\dfrac{1}{2} \div 3\dfrac{1}{5}$

13. $12\dfrac{4}{8} \div 4\dfrac{1}{2}$

14. $12\dfrac{4}{10} \div 3\dfrac{1}{3}$

15. $5\dfrac{1}{2} \div 1\dfrac{1}{8}$

16. $3\dfrac{5}{8} \div 2\dfrac{1}{2}$

17. $2\dfrac{3}{14} \div 9\dfrac{2}{7}$

18. $1\dfrac{7}{9} \div \dfrac{8}{11}$

19. $10\dfrac{6}{7} \div 7\dfrac{1}{2}$

20. $1\dfrac{9}{12} \div \dfrac{1}{12}$

Applications

1. A lab technician worked $45\dfrac{3}{4}$ hours in 5 days. He worked the same number of hours each day. How many hours a day did he work?

2. How many $\dfrac{1}{4}$ gram doses can be obtained from a $7\dfrac{1}{2}$ gram vial of medication?

3. The pharmacy technician's paycheck was for $1,123.85. If the technician worked $84\dfrac{1}{2}$ hours, what is the hourly rate of pay?

4. The nurse must give a patient 9 milligrams of a medication. If the tablets are 2 milligrams each, how many tablets are needed?

5. The pharmacy has 5 gram vials of medication. How many $\dfrac{1}{2}$ gram doses are available?

Fraction Formula

Follow these two setups:

To convert Celsius to Fahrenheit: $\left({}^\circ C \times \dfrac{9}{5} \right) + 32 = {}^\circ F$

To convert Fahrenheit to Celsius: $({}^\circ F - 32) \times \dfrac{5}{9} = {}^\circ C$

The decimal unit (Unit 3) will include the formula for handling temperature conversions using decimals.

Follow these steps to change a Fahrenheit temperature to a Celsius temperature:

Example $5{}^\circ C = \underline{\hspace{1cm}} {}^\circ F$

Step 1: Solve within the parentheses first, and then work left to right.

$$\left({}^\circ C \times \dfrac{9}{5} \right) + 32 = {}^\circ F$$

$$°C \times \frac{9}{5} \rightarrow \quad 5 \times \frac{9}{5} = \frac{45}{5} \qquad 5\overline{)45} = 9$$
$$\phantom{5\overline{)}}\underline{45}$$

Step 2: Add 32 to the step 1 answer to get the °C.

$$9 + 32 = 41 \ °F$$

> Fractions are used to convert between Celsius and Fahrenheit temperatures. Fractions are more accurate than decimals because there is no change in the numbers as a result of the rounding of decimals.

Practice
1. 20°C = _____ °F

2. 35°C = _____ °F

3. 25°C = _____ °F

4. 60°C = _____ °F

5. 40°C = _____ °F

6. 45°C = _____ °F

7. 80°C = _____ °F

8. 15°C = _____ °F

Follow these steps to change a Fahrenheit temperature to a Celsius temperature:

Example $122°F = \underline{\qquad} °C$

Step 1: Solve within the parenthesis first. $(°F - 32) \times \frac{5}{9} = °C$

$$°F - 32 = \underline{\qquad} \qquad \text{Subtract 32 from the}$$
$$122°F \qquad\qquad\quad \text{Fahrenheit temperature.}$$
$$\underline{-32}$$
$$90$$

Step 2: Multiply step 1 answer by $\frac{5}{9}$ to get the °C.

$$90 \times \frac{5}{9} = \frac{450}{9} \quad \text{Divide 450 by 9.}$$

$$\begin{array}{r} 50 \\ 9\overline{)450} \\ \underline{45\downarrow} \\ 00 \end{array}$$

So, 122°F is 50°C.

Practice

1. 104°F = _____ °C

2. 32°F = _____ °C

3. 50°F = _____ °C

4. 113°F = _____ °C

5. 59°F = _____ °C

6. 131°F = _____ °C

7. 86°F = _____ °C

8. 122°F = _____ °C

Some temperatures will require working with decimals. Additional practice will be provided in Unit 3: Decimals.

Complex Fractions

Complex fractions are used to help nurses and pharmacy technicians compute exact dosages. Complex fractions may also more efficiently solve difficult problems. A complex fraction is a fraction within a fraction.

Example

$$\frac{\frac{1}{4}}{6} \qquad \frac{\frac{3}{4}}{\frac{1}{100}}$$

These fraction lines should be viewed as a division sign.

Complex fractions are solved by using the rules of division. These examples become:

$$\frac{1}{4} \div 6 \rightarrow \frac{1}{4} \div \frac{6}{1} \rightarrow \frac{1}{4} \times \frac{1}{6} = \frac{1}{24}$$

$$\frac{3}{4} \div \frac{1}{100} \rightarrow \frac{3}{4} \div \frac{1}{100} \rightarrow \frac{3}{4} \times \frac{100}{1} = \frac{300}{4} \quad \text{Reduce to } \frac{75}{1} = 75$$

> Whole numbers require placing a 1 as a denominator prior to any division or multiplication of their digits.

Practice   Solve these complex fractions. Reduce to the lowest terms.

1. $\dfrac{\dfrac{3}{8}}{4}$

2. $\dfrac{\dfrac{1}{8}}{100}$

3. $\dfrac{\dfrac{1}{300}}{50}$

4. $\dfrac{40}{\dfrac{1}{25}}$

5. $\dfrac{\dfrac{1}{50}}{\dfrac{1}{60}}$

6. $\dfrac{\dfrac{3}{4}}{\dfrac{2}{3}}$

7. $\dfrac{\dfrac{1}{125}}{\dfrac{2}{200}}$

8. $\dfrac{\dfrac{1}{2}}{\dfrac{1}{4}}$

9. $\dfrac{\dfrac{1}{80}}{\dfrac{1}{75}}$

10. $\dfrac{\dfrac{1}{10}}{\dfrac{1}{100}}$

Dosage problems will also combine complex fractions with whole numbers and decimal numbers to compute the correct dosage. This work will be further covered in Unit 11: Dosage Calculations.

$$\dfrac{\dfrac{1}{300}}{\dfrac{1}{100}} \times 200$$

Example   These types of problems appear more difficult than they actually are. Group the work into sections so that it is manageable, and you can track your progress.

Step 1: Solve the complex fraction first by dividing it.

$$\frac{1}{300} \div \frac{1}{100} \rightarrow \frac{1}{300} \times \frac{100}{1} = \frac{100}{300} \rightarrow \text{Reduce to } \frac{1}{3}$$

Step 2: Next, rewrite the entire problem.

$$\frac{1}{3} \times 200 \qquad \text{Then work this portion of the problem.}$$

$$\frac{1}{3} \times \frac{200}{1} = \frac{200}{3} \quad \text{Reduce by dividing 200 by 3.}$$

The answer is $66\,^2/_3$. If the problem has a fraction it in, the answer may have a fraction in it. Do not convert this fraction to a decimal number.

Practice   Solve these problems.

1. $\dfrac{\frac{5}{8}}{\frac{1}{4}} \times 2$

2. $\dfrac{\frac{1}{200}}{\frac{1}{100}} \times 80$

3. $\dfrac{\frac{15}{500}}{\frac{1}{100}} \times 4$

4. $\dfrac{\frac{1}{125}}{\frac{1}{500}} \times 25$

5. $\dfrac{\frac{1}{3}}{\frac{1}{2}} \times 1\frac{1}{2}$

6. $\dfrac{\frac{1}{100}}{\frac{2}{25}} \times 10\frac{1}{4}$

FRACTION SELF-TEST

Reduce all answers to lowest terms.

1. A day has 24 hours. Six hours is what fractional part of the 24 hours?

2. Write two equivalent fractions for $\frac{1}{6}$.

3. Reduce $\frac{122}{11}$

4. $8\dfrac{1}{6} + 3\dfrac{3}{4}$

5. $52 - 12\dfrac{1}{5}$

6. $14\dfrac{1}{2} \times 2\dfrac{1}{8}$

7. $5\dfrac{2}{6} \div 12$

8. $77°\ F = \underline{\hspace{1cm}} °\ C$

9. Order from smallest to largest: $\dfrac{3}{8}, \dfrac{1}{3}, \dfrac{1}{4}, \dfrac{2}{12}$

10. Solve: $\dfrac{\frac{1}{4}}{\frac{1}{8}} \times 25$

11. The doctor orders grain $^1/_8$ of a medicine. The nurse has grain $^1/_6$ on hand in the medicine cabinet. Will the nurse give more or less of the dose on hand? _____

12. The physical therapist asks Mr. Smith to walk 20 minutes in one hour to improve his ambulation. What fractional part of an hour is Mr. Smith to exercise? _____

13. Among the fractions $^1/_3$, $^1/_5$, $^5/_8$, which one is equivalent to $^{15}/_{24}$? _____

14. On the dietitian's beverage tray, there are 16 filled six-ounce glasses. Four glasses contain prune juice and two glasses contain red wine. What fractional part of the glasses contains some beverage other than prune juice or red wine? Express the answer as a fraction. _____

15. Sally works in a nursery. Her job includes recording an accurate weight for each baby. One baby weighs $7\frac{1}{3}$ pounds, two babies weigh $6\frac{1}{2}$ pounds, and a fourth baby weighs $5\frac{7}{8}$ pounds. What is the current total weight of the babies? _____

Unit 3

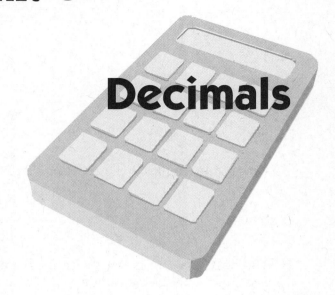

Decimals

Decimals are used every day in health care settings. Understanding the application of decimals provides a strong foundation for measurement conversions, the metric system, medication dosages, and general charting work. Most medication orders are written using the metric system, which relies on decimals.

A decimal represents a part or fraction of a whole number. Decimal numbers are parts of 10s, 100s, 1000s, and so on. In other words, decimals are multiples of ten. The decimal point (•) represents the boundary between whole numbers and decimal numbers.

Decimal Place Values								
whole numbers					decimal numbers			
thousands	hundreds	tens	ones	and	tenths	hundredths	thousandths	ten-thousandths	hundred-thousandths
	1	0	4	•	9	9			

Consider $104.99. We understand this number to be one hundred four dollars and ninety-nine cents. The decimal point is the *and* if we write the number in words.

Any number to the left of the decimal point is always a whole number and any number to the right of the decimal point is a decimal number. Without a whole number, a decimal number is always less than 1. So we understand that 0.89 and 0.123 are less than 1.

Health care workers include a zero to the left of the decimal point for any decimal that does not include a whole number. This signals the reader that the dose, measurement, or amount is less than 1. The zero also helps avoid errors caused by misreading a decimal number. This does not change the value of the number.

Examples   0.89 and 0.123

Decimal Place Values

whole numbers					**decimal numbers**			
thousands	hundreds	tens	ones	and	tenths	hundredths	thousandths	ten-thousandths	hundred-thousandths
		4	2	•	1	2	5		

Reading decimal numbers is simple if you follow these tips: To read decimal numbers, say the numbers from left to right as if they were whole numbers, then add the decimal place value.

42.125 → read as forty-two and one hundred twenty-five thousandths.

> Identify decimal numbers by looking for the words that end in "th" or "ths."

Write the decimals in words using this method:

1. 0.7

2. 0.89

3. 0.05

4. 4.3

5. 150.075

6. 34.009

7. 125.023

8. 47.9

9. 18.08

10. 0.126

Write the following words in decimal numbers:

1. two tenths

2. thirteen thousandths

3. three hundred and two thousandths

4. sixteen hundredths

5. six and three hundredths

To double-check your work, the final or last number should be placed in the place value spot of the words used to describe it. If it is hundredths, then the second decimal place must have a number in it.

Example

fifty-six thousandths

0.056

↑ thousandths place

Rounding Decimals

Decimals are rounded in health care to create manageable numbers. We may have a difficult time visualizing a number such as 14.39757. However, we can easily understand the number 14.4 or 14.40. Rounding to a specific decimal place is accomplished in the same way that whole numbers are rounded. In general, health care workers round decimal numbers to the nearest tenth or the nearest hundredth.

Example Round 1.75 to the nearest tenth.

Step 1: Underline the place to which you are rounding

1.7̲5

Step 2: Circle one number to the right of the underlined number. If the circled number is 5 or greater, add 1 to the underlined number, and drop all the numbers to the right of the changed number.

1.7̲5̄   → 1.8

If the circled number is less than 5, do not change the underlined number, and drop all the numbers to the right of that number.

Sometimes a health care worker will round to the tenths place value and the whole number will be affected.

Example   Round 4.97 to the nearest tenth.

Step 1:   4.<u>9</u>7

Step 2:   4.9⑦   4.9(Add 1 to 9) = 5.0 or 5

Practice   Round to the nearest tenth:

1. 6.74   6. 704.95

2. 249.86   7. 0.0943

3. 0.78   8. 349.37

4. 3.612   9. 9.89

5. 25.02   10. 0.087

Round to the nearest hundredth:

1. 17.327   6. $2,104.399

2. 0.975   7. 32.651

3. 4.8166   8. 9.27194

4. 0.0650   9. 46.085

5. 0.0074   10. 4.719

When and which place value to round to is a frequently asked question. General guidelines for rounding will be provided in Unit 11: Dosage Calculations.

Comparing Decimals

Comparing decimals is valuable in health occupations because many different pieces of equipment are used that may be in metric measurements. Decimals are part of the metric system, thus understanding them is necessary to determine which instrument or measurement is larger or smaller. Comparing decimals is a skill that is also useful in sorting and ordering inventory items by size.

To compare decimals, you will rely on your eyes rather than any specific math computation.

Example Which is larger: 0.081 or 0.28?

Step 1: Line the decimals up like buttons on a shirt. This will help make the decimal numbers appear to have the same number of decimal places.

0.081
0.28

Step 2: Add zeros to fill in the empty place values so that the numbers have the same number of places or digits.

0.081
0.280

Step 3: Disregard the decimal point for a moment and read the numbers as they are written from left to right, including the added zero place values.

0.081 → eighty-one
0.280 → two hundred eighty

So, 0.28 is larger than 0.081.

Practice Which decimal number is smaller?

1. 0.9 or 0.89

2. 0.025 or 0.5

3. 2.12 or 2.012

4. 0.4 or 0.04

5. 0.0033 or 0.03

Which is larger?

1. 0.0785 or 0.0195

2. 0.345 or 0.35

3. 0.5 or 0.055

4. 100.75 or 100.07

5. 0.0679 or 0.675

Using the same method, arrange the sets of numbers from largest to smallest:

1. 0.75, 7.5, 0.7, 7.075, 0.07

2. 0.01, 1.01, 10.01, 1.001

3. 0.5, 5.15, 5.55, 5.05, 0.05

4. 0.04, 0.004, 0.4, 0.044

Addition of Decimals

To add decimals, first line up the decimal points, then add. This might mean that the problem presented in a horizontal pattern may need to be rewritten in a vertical pattern.

A whole number always has a decimal point to the right side of the final number: $56 = 56$.

$$2.32 + 0.14 = ? \rightarrow \begin{array}{r} 2.32 \\ +0.14 \\ \hline 2.46 \end{array}$$

$$48 + 1.75 = \underline{\hspace{1cm}} \rightarrow \begin{array}{r} 48.00 \\ +\ 1.75 \\ \hline 49.75 \end{array}$$ ← Place a decimal point and fill the empty spaces with zeros.

Lining up the decimals is the first step in ensuring the correct answer for the addition of decimals.

$$2.46 + 0.005 + 1.3 = \underline{\hspace{1cm}} \rightarrow \begin{array}{r} 2.460 \\ 0.005 \\ +\ 1.300 \\ \hline 3.765 \end{array}$$ Fill the empty spaces with zeros.

Step 1: Line up the decimals. The order of the numbers to be added is unimportant.

Step 2: Add the numbers and bring the decimal point straight down.

Practice

1. $0.9 + 36 + 1.25$

2. $15.2 + 17.071 + 0.74$

3. $0.11 + 86 + 0.125$

4. $10.79 + 0.99 + 0.25$

5. $0.0096 + 50.24 + 39$

6. $0.849 + 1.6 + 56.3$

7. $14.28 + 16.24 + 97$

8. $0.75 + 23.87 + 124.07$

9. $13.75 + 0.001 + 200.53$

10. $35.01 + 76.02 + 0.0998$

Applications

1. A 25-year-old patient receives the following medication dosages daily: 1.5 milligrams, 2.25 milligrams, and 0.75 milligrams. What is his total dosage?

2. A child weighs 15.9 kilograms. The child has gained 0.9 and 1.5 kilograms during the past two months. What is the child's current weight?

3. Patient Smith receives 4 tablets of medication dosages daily: One tablet is 225 milligrams, two tablets are 0.125 milligrams each, and one tablet is 0.75 milligrams. What is the patient's total daily dosage of medication in milligrams?

4. One tablet is labeled 124 milligrams and another is labeled 0.5 milligrams. What is the total dosage of these two tablets?

5. A child measured 122 centimeters in a semiannual checkup with the doctor. What would be the child's height at the next office visit if the child grew by 2.54 centimeter?

Subtraction of Decimals

To subtract decimals, two steps are followed:

$$95.5 - 0.76 = \underline{\hspace{1cm}}$$

Step 1: Set the problem up vertically. Put the larger number or the number from which the second number is to be subtracted above, then line up the decimals.

$$\begin{array}{r} 95.50 \\ -\,0.76 \\ \hline \end{array}$$ ← Fill in the empty places with zeros.

Step 2: Subtract and then bring the decimal straight down.

$$9^4 5.^{14}5^10$$
$$-\ 0.\ \ 7\ \ 6$$
$$\overline{94.\ \ 7\ \ 4}$$

Practice

1. $3.4 - 2.68 =$

2. $69.4 - 5.04 =$

3. $15 - 0.935 =$

4. $0.48 - 0.3925 =$

5. $3.7 - 0.1987 =$

6. $12 - 1.932 =$

7. $0.2 - 0.025 =$

8. $14.47 - 0.3108 =$

9. $87.56 - 0.124 =$

10. $0.07 - 0.007 =$

Applications

1. A patient started with a 1 liter bag of IV solution. When the doctor checked in on the patient, the bag contained 0.35 liters of solution. How much solution was infused into the patient?

2. A bottle of medicine contains 30 milliliters. After withdrawing 2.25 milliliters for an injection, how many milliliters of medicine remain in the bottle?

3. A patient is to receive 4.25 milligrams of a drug daily. The patient has already received 2.75 milligrams. What is his remaining dosage in milligrams?

4. Patient B is on a low fat diet. He weighed 89.9 kilograms last month. This month he weighs 88.45 kilograms. How many kilograms has he lost?

5. A patient had a temperature of 101.4°F. If after medication, the patient's temperature is 99.6°F, what is the decrease in temperature?

Multiplication of Decimals

To multiply decimals, use the same process as in whole number multiplication. Do not line up the decimals. The decimal places are counted, not aligned in decimal multiplication.

Example

$$4.75 \times .4$$

Step 1: Write the problem vertically.

$$
\begin{array}{r}
4.75 \\
\times \ .4 \\
\hline
\end{array}
$$

Step 2: Multiply the numbers.

$$
\begin{array}{r}
4.75 \\
\times \quad .4 \\
\hline
1900
\end{array}
$$

Step 3: Count the total number of decimal places in the two numbers multiplied together. Count these places from the right in to the left. Then begin at the right of the answer and count over the same number of places and place the decimal point.

$$
\begin{array}{l}
4.75 \\
\quad \cup\cup \ 2 \ \text{places} \\
0.4 \\
\quad \cup \ 1 \ \text{place} \\
\hline
1.900 \\
\quad \cup\cup\cup
\end{array}
$$

Place the decimal point three places from the right. The extra zeros are dropped unless they serve a particular purpose, such as place holders for money in dollar figures.

$$
\begin{array}{ll}
17.750 & \rightarrow 17.75 \\
205.12600 & \rightarrow 205.126 \\
\$12.00 & \rightarrow \$12.00
\end{array}
$$

Practice   Set up multiplication problems vertically:

1. 4.2×3

2. 9.3×7

3. 21×1.6

4. 465×0.3

5. 9.17×14

6. 0.985×50

7. 6.74×0.12

8. 3.190×0.56

9. 0.278×1.7

10. 4.79×2.2

11. 0.08×0.03

12. 5.6×0.39

13. 5.175×29.2

14. $3,764 \times 13.75$

15. 9.708×0.17

16. 114.6×22.6

17. 190.8×0.04

18. 827.9×1.9

19. 574×12.095

20. 0.135×73.7

21. 53.9×24.9

22. 204.7×13.87

23. 0.347×28.95

24. 94.13×32.09

Applications

1. Village Center health care workers' earnings start at $10.52 an hour. If the employees work 40 hours per week, what is the minimum amount that each worker could earn in a week?

2. One mile has 1.6 kilometers. How many kilometers are in 35.5 miles?

3. Sheila earns $13.05 an hour. If she works 124 hours in August, what are her gross earnings for the month?

4. One kilogram equals 2.2 pounds. If patient A weighs 79.5 kilograms, what is his weight in pounds?

5. The recreation department is making placemats. The cost of materials for each placemat is $1.28. The activity director is estimating the cost of materials for 100 placemats. What is the estimated budget needed for this project?

Division of Decimals

To divide decimals, one needs to place the decimal point first, then divide the numbers. Once the decimal point is placed, it is not moved. Students have a tendency to want to move the decimal point once the division process is underway; the result is an error in decimal placement.

Follow the steps below to divide a number that has a decimal in the dividend:

Step 1: Move the decimal point straight up to the same place in the quotient. Place the decimal point and then divide the numbers.

$$6\overline{)2.58}$$

Step 2: Divide, adding a zero in front of all decimal numbers that do not include a whole number.

$$
\begin{array}{r}
0.43 \\
6\overline{)2.58} \\
\underline{2\,4} \\
18 \\
\underline{18} \\
0
\end{array}
$$

Practice

1. $19\overline{)11.97}$

2. $5\overline{)67.75}$

3. $2\overline{)0.464}$

4. $21\overline{)9.03}$

5. $12\overline{)1.44}$

6. $4\overline{)68.4}$

7. $32\overline{)1676.8}$

8. $17\overline{)51.17}$

9. $25\overline{)75.50}$

10. $34\overline{)2603.72}$

Zeros as Placeholders in Decimal Division

Health care students may need some practice in dividing decimals that involve zeros in the quotient. This is one area where errors are commonly made. To avoid this situation, recall that after a number has been brought down from the dividend, the divisor must be applied to that number. Place the decimal point and then divide the number. If the divisor does not go into the dividend, then a zero must be placed in the quotient. Use a zero to hold a space.

Example

$$
\begin{array}{r}
2.405 \\
14\overline{)33.67} \\
28\downarrow \\
\hline
56 \\
56\downarrow \\
\hline
07 \\
0\downarrow \\
\hline
70 \\
70 \\
\hline
0
\end{array}
$$

Because 14 cannot go into 7, place a zero in the quotient.

Setup Tip

Remember in division problem setup

$475 \div 4.5 =$

$\nearrow \quad \longrightarrow \quad$ *$4.5\overline{)475}$

*The last number in the problem divides into the first number.

To divide a decimal number by a decimal number, change the divisor to a whole number by moving the decimal point to the right. Then move the decimal point in the dividend the same number of places. Use zeros as placeholders if needed. Then place the decimal point and divide.

For example, $0.42\overline{)0.6216}$

Step 1: Move the decimal $0.42\overline{)0.6216}$ Rewrite → $42\overline{)62.16}$

Step 2: Divide $42\overline{)62.16}$

Practice

1. 530 ÷ 0.5

2. 0.081 ÷ 9

3. 66.56 ÷ 32

4. 0.022 ÷ 11

5. 3.297 ÷ 3

6. 0.6250 ÷ 5

7. 183.96 ÷ 6

8. 6.030 ÷ 3

9. 0.18891 ÷ 0.9

10. 12.24 ÷ 4

Additional Practice

1. $0.5\overline{)2.65}$

2. $0.04\overline{)6.48}$

3. $2.6\overline{)0.104}$

4. $0.55\overline{)141.35}$

5. $3.8\overline{)5.282}$

6. $0.7\overline{)78.75}$

7. $0.02\overline{)8.078}$

8. $0.3\overline{)4.608}$

Simplified Multiplication and Division of Decimals

Using the shortcuts of simplified multiplication and division can save time in working with decimals. In health-care fields, this shortcut is important to your work in metrics and in efficiently working longer problems.

This shortcut only works with multiples of ten: 10, 100, 1,000, etc. The process is straightforward. To multiply, move the decimal point to the right. To divide, move the decimal point to the left. The number of spaces depends on which multiple you are working with. Look at the number of zeros included in the multiple, then move the decimal in either direction depending on the operation: multiplication or division, the same number of spaces and the number of zeros.

Simplified Multiplication

To multiply by 10, locate the decimal point and move it to the right by one place.

To multiply by 100, locate the decimal point and move it to the right by two places.

To multiply by 1,000, locate the decimal point and move it to the right by three places.

Whole numbers have their decimal places to the far right of the last digit: $9 = 9., 75 = 75., 125 = 125.$

Example

$$4.5 \times 10 = 45 \qquad 4.5$$
$$4.5 = 45 \qquad \underline{\times \ 10}$$
$$\cup \qquad\qquad 45.0 \quad \text{(The Zero is dropped.)}$$

Note that the answer is the same if the problem is worked the long way. Sometimes zeros must be added as placeholders.

In simplified multiplication locate the decimal point, count the zeros in the divisor and move the decimal point the same number of places to the right.

Example Zeros must fill the spaces if needed.

$$34.7 \times 1000 = \underline{\qquad}$$
$$34.7\,0\,0 =$$
$$\cup\cup\cup \rightarrow 34,700$$

Practice
1. 13.5×10
2. 4.56×100
3. 125.75×10
4. $1,000 \times 45.3$

5. 0.06×100

6. 0.234×10

7. $12.67 \times 1,000$

8. 0.975×100

9. $0.476 \times 1,000$

10. 87×10

11. 1.345×10

12. $98.345 \times 1,000$

13. 1.009×10

14. 32.901×100

15. $23.850 \times 1,000$

Simplified Division

To divide by 10, locate the decimal point and move it to the left by one place.

To divide by 100, locate the decimal point and move it to the left by two places.

To divide by 1,000, locate the decimal point and move it to the left by three places.

In simplified division, locate the decimal point, count the zeros in the divisor and move the decimal point the same number of places to the left.

Example $9.5 \div 10 =$ _____ $0.75 \div 100 =$ _____
9.5   0 0 0.75 $\rightarrow$ 0.0075   Zeros must be used to fill
$\cup \rightarrow 0.95$ $\cup\cup$ in places if needed.

Practice   1. $12.9 \div 10$

2. $45.56 \div 100$

3. $125 \div 10$

4. $98.762 \div 1,000$

5. $0.25 \div 10$

6. $176.5 \div 100$

7. $15.8 \div 100$

8. $3,234 \div 10$

9. $32.50 \div 100$

10. $0.09 \div 10$

11. $10,010 \div 1,000$

12. $9,765 \div 1,000$

13. $3.076 \div 100$

14. $429.6 \div 1,000$

15. $10.275 \div 100$

Applications   1. A nursing student spends $379.50 for textbooks. If the student purchases six textbooks, what is the average cost of each book?

2. A patient's goal is to lose 24.6 pounds. The doctor wants the patient to lose these pounds slowly, over a twelve-month period. How many pounds should the patient attempt to lose each month?

3. Doctor Brown prescribed a medication dosage of 4.5 grams. How many 1.5 grams tablets need to be administered?

4. The dietitian serves a protein dish at three meals. If the total daily grams of protein are 225.9 grams, assuming that the grams are equally divided for the three meals a day, what is the average meal's grams of protein?

5. Bob made $131.20 in 5 hours. What is his hourly wage?

Changing Decimals to Fractions

It is important to be able to convert between number systems so that you are comfortable with comparing sizes of items or quantities of supplies. Changing decimals to fractions requires the use of decimal places and placing the numbers in fractions that represent the very same numbers.

Example Convert 0.457 to a fraction.

Step 1: To convert a decimal to a fraction, count the number of decimal places in the decimal number.

$$0.4\,5\,7 \qquad \text{Three decimal places means thousandths in decimal numbers.}$$

Step 2: Write the number 457 as the numerator and 1,000 as the denominator.

$$\frac{457}{1,000}$$

Step 3: Reduce if necessary $\frac{457}{1,000}$ cannot be reduced. The answer is $\frac{457}{1,000}$.

Example Convert 2.75 to a fraction.

Step 1: Place 2 as the whole number. Your answer is going to be a mixed number because there is a whole number. Count the decimal places in $.7\,5$ = two places.

$$2\ \underline{}$$

Step 2: Write 75 as the numerator and 100 as the denominator.

$$2\frac{75}{100}$$

Step 3: Reduce the fraction to $2\frac{3}{4}$ because

$$\frac{75}{100} = \frac{\cancel{25} \times 3}{\cancel{25} \times 4} \rightarrow \frac{3}{4}$$

The answer is $2\frac{3}{4}$.

Practice Convert the decimals to fractions:

1. 0.04

2. 0.025

3. 6.25

4. 1.78

5. 225.05

6. 10.5

7. 7.75

8. 0.08

9. 9.3

10. 100.46

Changing Fractions to Decimals

To change fractions to decimals, divide the denominator into the numerator. Critical to the success of this division is the placement of the decimal point. Once it is placed, do not move it.

Example Change $^3/_4$ to a decimal. Divide the denominator into the numerator. Place a decimal point after 3 and also in the quotient. Then add a zero after 3 and divide. Add zeros as needed to continue the division process.

$$\begin{array}{r} .75 \\ 4\overline{)3.0} \\ 28\downarrow \\ \hline 20 \\ 20 \\ \hline 0 \end{array}$$

Example Change $^1/_3$ into a decimal. Divide 3 into 1. Place the decimal point. Add zeros as needed to continue division. The division may not come out evenly but rather begin to repeat itself. After two places, make the remainder into a fraction by putting the remaining number over the divisor.

$$\begin{array}{r} .33\frac{1}{3} \\ 3\overline{)1.0} \\ 9\downarrow \\ \hline 10 \\ 9 \\ \hline 1 \end{array}$$

> When the decimal answer is a number like 0.50, drop the final zero so that the answer is 0.5.

Practice   1. $\dfrac{1}{2}$

2. $\dfrac{3}{5}$

3. $\dfrac{7}{8}$

4. $\dfrac{1}{6}$

5. $\dfrac{6}{25}$

6. $\dfrac{5}{12}$

7. $\dfrac{3}{15}$

8. $\dfrac{7}{10}$

9. $\dfrac{5}{6}$

10. $\dfrac{3}{18}$

Temperature Conversions with Decimals

The following temperature conversions include decimals. Round the decimal numbers in temperatures to the nearest tenth place. The temperature conversion used in Unit 2: Fractions, relied on fractions. The same fraction method can be converted into a decimal method. In deciding which method to use, select the method of fractions or decimals based on your strongest skill. Then consistently use that conversion formula.

Decimal Conversion Formula

To convert Celsius to Fahrenheit, $(°C \times 1.8) + 32 = °F$

To convert Fahrenheit to Celsius, $(°F - 32) \div 1.8 = °C$

Example   To convert from Celsius to Fahrenheit

$$41°C = \underline{\hspace{1cm}} °F$$

Step 1: Solve the parentheses first, and then work left to right. Multiply the Celsius temperature by 1.8. The number 1.8 is the decimal form of $9/5$.

$$\begin{array}{r} 41 \\ \times\ 1.8 \\ \hline 328 \\ 41 \\ \hline 73.8 \end{array}$$

Step 2: Add 32 to the step 1 answer.

$$\begin{array}{r} 73.8 \\ +\ 32 \\ \hline 105.8 \end{array}$$

The answer is 105.8°F.

To convert from Fahrenheit to Celsius

Step 1: Subtract the 32 from the Fahrenheit temperature.

$$\begin{array}{r} 107.6 \\ -\ 32 \\ \hline 75.6 \end{array}$$

Step 2: Divide the step 1 answer by 1.8.

$$\rightarrow 1.8\overline{)75.6} \rightarrow \quad \begin{array}{r} 42. \\ 18\overline{)756.} \\ 72 \\ \hline 36 \\ 36 \\ \hline 0 \end{array}$$

The answer is 42°C.

Practice   1. 34°C = _____ °F

2. 46.6°F = _____ °C

3. 107°C = _____ °F

4. 101.5°F = _____ °C

5. 42°C = _____ °F

6. 40°F = _____ °C

7. 100.4°F = _____ °C

8. $69°C =$ _____ $°F$

9. $12°C =$ _____ $°F$

10. $105.8°F =$ _____ $°C$

Solving Mixed Fraction and Decimal Problems

Sometimes problems will include both fractions and decimals. The very same processes of solving the problems are still needed; however, the order of handling the parts of the problem may vary. Group the math computations inside the problem to best manage the separate operations.

> If the problem has a complex fraction multiplied by a decimal number, work the complex fraction first. Then complete the decimal multiplication.

Example

$$\frac{\frac{1}{2}}{\frac{1}{5}} \times 2.2 =$$

Step 1:

$$\frac{1}{2} \div \frac{1}{5} \rightarrow \frac{1}{2} \times \frac{5}{1} = \frac{5}{2}$$

Reduce to $2\frac{1}{2}$. Make the $\frac{1}{2}$ into .5 so that the multiplication is easy. So by first working the complex fraction, the answer is 2.5.

Step 2: Multiply 2.5×2.2.

$$\begin{array}{r} 2.5 \\ \times\ 2.2 \\ \hline 50 \\ 50 \\ \hline 5.50 \end{array}$$

The answer to this mixed problem is 5.5.

> If the problem includes a decimal number, solve the decimals by first multiplying straight across, then complete the process by dividing that answer by the denominator. This allows for the division of decimals only once, and it saves time.

Example $\dfrac{0.25}{0.5} \times 1.5$

Step 1: Multiply 0.25×1.5.

$$
\begin{array}{r}
0.25 \\
\times\ 1.5 \\
\hline
125 \\
25 \\
\hline
0.375
\end{array}
$$

Step 2: Divide 0.375 by 0.5.

$0.5\overline{)0.375}$

$$
\begin{array}{r}
0.75 \\
0.5\overline{)0.375} \\
0.35 \\
\hline
0025 \\
0025 \\
\hline
0
\end{array}
$$

The answer is 0.75.

Practice

1. $\dfrac{\frac{1}{200}}{\frac{1}{100}} \times 4.4$

2. $\dfrac{0.8}{0.64} \times 4.5$

3. $\dfrac{\frac{3}{4}}{\frac{1}{4}} \times 2.5$

4. $\dfrac{0.75}{0.15} \times 1.5$

5. $\dfrac{0.002}{0.125} \times 10.5$

6. $\dfrac{\frac{1}{12}}{\frac{1}{6}} \times 3.6$

7. $\dfrac{0.005}{0.01} \times 15.35$

8. $\dfrac{7\frac{1}{2}}{1\frac{1}{2}} \times 5.4$

DECIMAL SELF-TEST

1. Write in words: 0.045

2. What is the sum of 1.7, 19, 0.25, and 0.8?

3. $17 - 0.075$

4. 4.5×1.009

5. $18.04 \div 0.2$

6. Round to the nearest hundredth: 978.735

7. Order these decimals from largest to smallest: 0.81, 0.080, 0.018, 8.018.

8. 10.009×100

9. A child receives 0.5 milligrams of a drug 4 times a day. How many milligrams is the child's daily dose?

10. A patient receives 2.25 grams of a medication daily. Tablets come in 0.75 gram dosages. How many tablets does the patient take daily?

11. Convert this decimal to a fraction: 0.125

12. Convert this fraction to a decimal: $\dfrac{13}{50}$

13. Convert this fraction to a decimal: $3\dfrac{5}{8}$

14. Convert 103° Fahrenheit to °Celsius.

15. Solve:

$$\dfrac{0.136}{0.2} \times 2.5$$

Unit 4

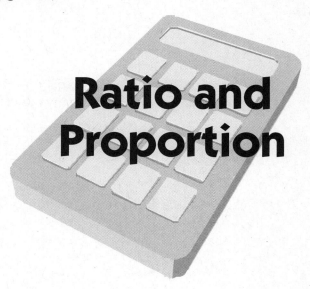

Ratio and Proportion

Ratio

A ratio is used to show a relationship between two numbers. These numbers are separated by a colon (:) as in 3 : 4. Ratios may be presented in three formats that provide the setup for solving proportions.

   a. 3 : 4

   b. $\frac{3}{4}$

   c. 3 is to 4

The relationship can represent something as simple as the 1 : 3 ratio commonly used to mix frozen juices. We use 1 can of frozen juice concentrate to 3 cans of water. Ratios are fractions that represent a part-to-whole relationship. Ratios are always reduced to their lowest form. For example, 8 hours of sleep to 24 hours in a day

$$8 : 24 \rightarrow \frac{8}{24} \quad \frac{8 \times 1}{8 \times 3} = \frac{1}{3}, \quad \text{so the ratio is 1 : 3.}$$

Write the following relationships as ratios using a colon. Reduce to the lowest terms, if necessary.

1. 5 days out of 7 days

2. eight teeth out of thirty-two teeth

3. 3 students out of 15 students

4. 16 scalpels to 45 syringes

5. 7 inlays to 14 crowns

Simplifying ratios is an important skill. To simplify a ratio, divide the first number by the second.

For example, simplify the following ratio: $4\frac{1}{2} : 6$

$$4\frac{1}{2} \div 6 \rightarrow \frac{9}{2} \div \frac{6}{1} \rightarrow \frac{9}{2} \times \frac{1}{6} = \frac{9}{12} \rightarrow \frac{3 \times 3}{3 \times 4} = \frac{3}{4}$$ which becomes $3:4$ as a simplified ratio.

The answer is $3:4$.

For example, simplify the following ratio: $11\frac{1}{4}$

Convert the mixed number into an improper fraction, then reduce if necessary.

$$11\frac{1}{4} \rightarrow 11 \times 4 + 1 = 45 \rightarrow \frac{45}{4} = 45:4$$

The answer is $45:4$.

Simplify the following ratios. Write each answer as a ratio.

1. $45 : 1\frac{2}{3}$ = _____

2. $\frac{120}{100} : 12$ = _____

3. $15 : \frac{3}{4}$ = _____

4. $\frac{1}{3} : 45$ = _____

5. $0.8 : \frac{2}{5}$ = _____

6. $\frac{1}{2} : \frac{1}{8}$ = _____

7. $4\frac{1}{3} : 7$ = _____

8. $0.875 : \frac{1}{4}$ = _____

9. $2\frac{1}{2}$ = _____

10. $\frac{2}{3} : 0.33$ = _____

Proportion

Proportions can be applied to almost every health care profession in one way or another. In addition to on-the-job applications, proportions provide a simple and quick method for solving many everyday math problems such as measurement conversions, recipe conversions for increasing or decreasing the amounts of ingredients, and map mileage.

Proportions are *two or more equivalent ratios or fractions*. The terms of the first ratio/fraction have the same relationship of part to whole as the second ratio/fraction.

Example
$$\frac{3}{4} = \frac{15}{20} \text{ or } 3:4::15:20$$

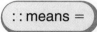 :: means =

Test the two ratios/fractions to see whether they are equivalent by multiplying diagonally (cross multiply).

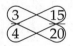 $4 \times 15 = 60$ and $3 \times 20 = 60$. This is a proportion.

If the two numbers that are diagonal result in the same answer when they are multiplied, you are working with a proportion.

Proportions are powerful tools in health care. You can rely on them for solving a majority of your math conversions and problems. Check to see if the following ratios are proportions:

Are these ratios proportions?

1. $5:2 = 4:1$ _____ Yes   _____ No

2. $16:15 = 8:7$ _____ Yes   _____ No

3. $40:30 = 4:3$ _____ Yes   _____ No

4. $10:16 = 5:8$ _____ Yes   _____ No

5. $100:1 = 50:2$ _____ Yes   _____ No

Solving for *x*

The ratio and proportion method of solving for *x* is done in two steps.

Step 1: Set the problems up like fractions. If units of measure such as inches and feet are given, place inches across from inches and feet across from feet. Then cross multiply (diagonally) the two numbers. Set the ratios up like fractions using a vertical line.

$$\frac{3}{4} = \frac{?}{16} \quad 3 \times 16 = 48$$

Step 2:   Divide the answer from step 1 by the remaining number.

$$
\begin{array}{r}
12 \\
4\overline{)48} \\
4\downarrow \\
\hline
8 \\
8 \\
\hline
\end{array}
$$

The quotient 12 is the answer to ? or x. This method is an easy way to find the answers for measurement conversions, dosage conversions, and math questions that provide part but not all of the information.

Practice   Solve for x or ?

1. $20 : 40 = x : 15$

2. $x : 1 = 5 : 10$

3. $4 : 8 = 8 : x$

4. $7 : x = 21 : 24$

5. $3 : 9 = ? : 81$

6. $13 : 39 = 1 : ?$

7. $2 : 11 = ? : 77$

8. $x : 125 = 5 : 25$

9. $2 : 26 = 4 : ?$

10. $1 : x = 5 : 200$

Using ratios is often the simplest method of solving other health care math problems, such as dosage calculations and measurement problems.

Example   Zoe weighs 35 pounds. The doctor ordered a drug that relies on milligrams of medication to kilograms of body weight. The pharmacy technician will need to convert pounds to kilograms. By using the ratio of 1 kilogram to 2.2 pounds, the answer is quickly computed.

$$
\begin{array}{cc}
\textit{known} & \textit{unknown} \\
\dfrac{1 \text{ kilogram}}{2.2 \text{ pounds}} & \dfrac{?}{35 \text{ pounds}}
\end{array}
$$

Step 1:   Multiply the numbers diagonally.

$$1 \times 35 = 35$$

Step 2:   Divide 35 by 2.2. The answer is 15.9 kilograms.

So 35 pounds equals 15.9 kilograms.

Example   How many pounds are in 24 ounces?
Set the problem up by placing what you know on the left side of the equation and what you do not know on the right. If you set up all your problems with the known on the left and the unknown on the right, you will have less information for the brain to process because the pattern will be familiar to you.

known	unknown
1 pound	? pounds
16 ounces	24 ounces

Step 1: $1 \times 24 = 24$

Step 2: $24 \div 16 = 1.5$

The answer is $1\frac{1}{2}$ pounds or 1.5 pounds.
An answer for a ratio may have a decimal or a fraction in it.

Example   Bob is 176 centimeters (cm) tall. How tall is he in inches? Round the answer to the nearest tenth.

known	unknown
1 inch	? inches
2.54 cm	176 cm

Step 1: $1 \times 176 = 176$

Step 2: $176 \div 2.54 = 69.29$

Rounded to the nearest tenth.
The answer is 69.3 inches.

$$
\begin{array}{r}
69.29 \\
254)\overline{17600} \\
1524\downarrow \\
\overline{2360} \\
2286\downarrow \\
\overline{740} \\
508\downarrow \\
\overline{2320} \\
2286 \\
\overline{34}
\end{array}
$$

Some basic guidelines need to be followed for formatting answers in measurement conversions:

If the answer is in feet, yards, cups, pints, quarts, gallons, teaspoons, tablespoons, or pounds, use fractions if there is a remainder.

If the answer is in kilograms, milliliters, or money amounts, use decimals. The correct format ensures correct answers.

Approximate Equivalents

1 inch	= 2.54 centimeters	1 cup	= 8 ounces
1 foot	= 12 inches	1 pint	= 500 milliliters
1 yard	= 3 feet	1 quart	= 32 ounces
1 pound	= 16 ounces	1 quart	= 1,000 milliliters
1 kilogram	= 2.2 pounds		
1 tablespoon	= 3 teaspoons	1 fluid ounce	= 30 milliliters
1 quart	= 2 pints	1 teaspoon	= 5 milliliters
1 gallon	= 4 quarts	1 fluid ounce	= 2 tablespoons

Notice that the conversions are set up so that the unit (1) elements are all on the left and that these will be placed on the top of the known part of the ratio and proportion equation. This simplifies the learning process, expedites learning, and helps recall of these conversions.

Practice   Because inches are rounded to the nearest tenth, go to the hundredth place and then stop multiplying. At that point, you will have enough information to round to the nearest tenth.

Using this ratio and proportion setup, solve the following conversions.

$$\frac{known}{\rule{2cm}{0.4pt}} = \frac{unknown}{\rule{2cm}{0.4pt}}$$

Set up these conversions using ratios and proportions.

1. 23 feet = _____ yards → $\dfrac{1\,yd}{3\,ft} = \dfrac{?}{23\,ft}$

2. 12 quarts = _____ gallons

3. 4 quarts = _____ pints

4. 4 pints = _____ cups

5. 3 tablespoons = _____ teaspoons

6. $2\frac{1}{2}$ quarts = _____ milliliters

7. $\frac{1}{2}$ cup = _____ ounces

8. 1 injection at $29.50 = 3 injections at _____

9. $3\frac{1}{2}$ pounds = _____ ounces

10. 3 medicine cups = _____ milliliters

   (One medicine cup equals 1 fluid ounce)

11. 12.5 mL = _____ teaspoons

12. 5 fluid ounces = _____ tablespoons

13. _____ tablespoons = 15 teaspoons

14. 64 ounces = _____ cups

15. 750 milliliters = _____ pints

16. 48 inches = _____ feet

17. 5 pounds = _____ ounces

18. _____ quarts = 5,000 milliliters

29. _____ kilograms = 11 pounds

20. $3\frac{1}{2}$ cups = _____ ounces

More practice with conversions of measurements between systems and with multiple steps in conversions will be given in Unit 6: Combined Applications.

Word Problems Using Proportions

When solving word problems involving proportions, follow these two basic steps:

Step 1: Set the problem up so that the same type of elements are directly across from one another.

Example   If 12 eggs cost $1.49, how much do 18 eggs cost?

$$\frac{\text{Eggs}}{\text{Cost}} = \frac{\text{Eggs}}{\text{Cost}} \rightarrow \frac{12\,\text{eggs}}{\$1.49} = \frac{18\,\text{eggs}}{\$?}$$

Step 2: Ensure that the story problem is understood, then place the known information on the left side of the proportion and the unknown on the right. By doing so, you will not switch the ratio relationships, but rather rely on the known part to whole relationships.

1. A caplet contains 325 milligrams of medication. How many caplets contain 975 milligrams of medication?

2. If a dose of 100 milligrams is contained in 4 cubic centimeters, how many cubic centimeters are in 40 milligrams?

3. If 35 grams of pure drug are contained in 150 milliliters, how many grams are contained in 75 milliliters?

4. Two tablets of ulcer medication contain 350 milligrams of medication. How many milligrams are in twelve tablets?

5. If 1 kilogram equals 2.2 pounds, how many kilograms are in 61.6 pounds?

Solving for X in More Complex Problems Using Proportion

Decimals and fractions may appear in your proportion problems. Although the numbers may be visually distracting, the *very* same principles apply.

Example $0.25 \ \text{mg} : 0.8 \ \text{mL} = 0.125 \ \text{mg} : x \ \text{mL}$

Step 1: Place mg across from mg and mL across from mL. Place the known information on the left side of the equation and the unknown on the right.

$$\frac{\overset{known}{0.25\ mg}}{0.8\ mL}\quad\frac{\overset{unknown}{0.125\ mg}}{x\ mL}$$

Cross multiply $0.8 \times 0.125\ mg = 0.1$.

Step 2: $0.1 \div 0.25 = 0.4\ mL$

Example

$$\frac{1}{8} : \frac{1}{2} :: 1 : x$$

Step 1: Set up and cross multiply. Multiply $\frac{1}{2} \times 1 = \frac{1}{2}$.

$$\frac{1/8}{1/2} = \frac{1}{x}$$

Step 2: Divide $\frac{1}{2}$ by $\frac{1}{8}$.

$$\frac{1}{2} \div \frac{1}{8} \rightarrow \frac{1}{2} \times \frac{8}{1} = \frac{8}{2}, \quad \text{which is reduced to 4.}$$

Sometimes you will find that medical dosages have both fractions and decimals in the problems. Analyze the situation and convert the numbers into the same system. As a general rule, fractions are always more accurate for calculating than decimals because some decimal numbers have repeating digits, which create variable answers.

Example

$$\frac{1}{16} : 1.6 :: \frac{1}{8} x$$

Step 1: Convert 1.6 into a fraction. So $1.6 = 1\frac{6}{10}$. Then multiply $1\frac{6}{10} \times \frac{1}{8} = \frac{2}{10}$

$$\frac{1/16}{1\frac{6}{10}} = \frac{1/8}{x} \qquad 1\frac{6}{10} \times \frac{1}{8} = \frac{16}{10} \times \frac{1}{8} = \frac{16}{80} \text{ or } \frac{2}{10}$$

Step 2: Divide $\frac{2}{10}$ by $\frac{1}{16}$.

$$\frac{2}{10} \div \frac{1}{16} \rightarrow \frac{2}{10} \times \frac{16}{1} = \frac{32}{10} \quad \text{Reduced to } 3\frac{2}{10} \rightarrow 3\frac{1}{5}.$$

Practice Include a unit of measure in your answer. Round any partial unit to the nearest tenth.

> Tablets can be divided if they are scored; use $\frac{1}{2}$ not 0.5

1. $1.5\ mg : 2\ caps = 4.5\ mg : x\ caps$

2. $8\ mg : 2.5\ mL = 4\ mg : x\ mL$

3. $12.5 \text{ mg} : 5 \text{ mL} = 24 \text{ mg} : x \text{ mL}$

4. $0.3 \text{ mg} : 1 \text{ tab} = 6 \text{ mg} : x \text{ tabs}$

5. $\text{grains } \dfrac{1}{4} : 15 \text{ mg} = \text{grains ? } : 60 \text{ mg}$

6. $x \text{ mg} : \dfrac{1}{2} \text{ tab} = 6 \text{ mg} : 4 \text{ tabs}$

7. $\text{grains } \dfrac{1}{100} : 2 \text{ mL} = \text{grains } \dfrac{1}{15c} : x \text{ mL}$

8. $600 \text{ mg} : 1 \text{ cap} = x \text{ mg} : 2 \text{ caps}$

9. $1000 \text{ units} : 1 \text{ mL} = 2400 \text{ units} : x \text{ mL}$

10. $1 \text{ tab} : 0.1 \text{ mg} = x \text{ tabs} : 0.15 \text{ mg}$

11. A drug comes in 100 milligram tablets. If the doctor orders 150 milligrams daily, how many tablets should the patient receive daily?

12. A medical chart states that the patient weighs 78.4 kilograms. What is the patient's weight in pounds? Round to the nearest tenth.

Nutritional Application of Proportions

Carbohydrates, fats, and protein provide fuel factors for our bodies. The factors are easily applied by using proportions to solve for the unknown.

Carbohydrates	→ 4 calories per 1 gram
Fats	→ 9 calories per 1 gram
Proteins	→ 4 calories per 1 gram

Example 400 carbohydrate calories = _____ grams

$$\underset{\textit{known}}{\dfrac{1 \text{ gram}}{4 \text{ calories}}} \qquad \underset{\textit{unknown}}{\dfrac{? \text{ grams}}{400 \text{ calories}}}$$

Step 1: Multiply diagonally.

$$1 \times 400 = 400$$

Step 2: Divide answer from step 1 (400) by the remaining number in the equation (4).

$$\begin{array}{r} 100 \\ 4\overline{)400} \\ \underline{4} \\ 00 \end{array}$$

So 400 carbohydrate calories are available in 100 grams of carbohydrates.

Use proportion to solve the following problems:

1. 81 calories of fat = _____ grams

2. 120 calories of protein = _____ grams

3. 36 calories of carbohydrate = _____ grams

4. 145 calories of carbohydrate = _____ grams

5. _____ calories in 12 grams of protein

6. _____ calories in 99 grams of fat

7. _____ calories in 328 grams of carbohydrate

8. _____ calories in 2450 grams of protein

Proportion is also useful in solving measurement problems that have to do with amounts of sodium, calories, fat, and protein in food or an amount in a drug dosage. The proportion will use the information in a scenario to solve for the unknown quantities in a specific amount.

Example If one glass of milk contains 280 milligrams of calcium, how much calcium is in $1\frac{1}{2}$ glasses of milk?

$$\frac{1\ \text{glass}}{280\ \text{milligrams}} = \frac{1\frac{1}{2}\ \text{glasses}}{?\ \text{milligrams}}$$

$$280 \times 1\frac{1}{2} = 420\ \text{mg of calcium}$$

1. One-half cup of baked beans contains 430 milligrams of sodium. How many milligrams of sodium are there in $\frac{3}{4}$ cup of baked beans?

2. Baked beans contain 33 grams of carbohydrates in a $\frac{1}{2}$ cup serving. How many milligrams of carbohydrates are in three $\frac{1}{2}$ cup servings?

3. A $\frac{1}{2}$ cup serving of fruit cocktail contains 55 milligrams of potassium. How many milligrams of potassium are in 2 cups of fruit cocktail?

4. If $\frac{1}{2}$ cup of fruit cocktail contains 13 grams of sugar, then $1\frac{1}{4}$ cup of fruit cocktail contains how many grams of sugar?

5. Old-fashioned oatmeal contains 27 grams of carbohydrates per $\frac{1}{2}$ cup of dry oats. How many grams of carbohydrates are available in $2\frac{1}{4}$ cups of the dry oats?

Practice with Food Labels

Carefully read the label and then use the information from the label to solve each question.

Albert's Tomato Soup

Nutrition facts	Amount/serving %DV*		Amount/serving %DV*	
Serving size ½ cup (120 ml)	Total fat 0 g	0%	Total carbohydrates 20 g	7%
Condensed soup	Saturated fat 0 g	0%	Fiber 1 g	4%
Servings about 2.5	Cholesterol 0 mg	0%	Sugars 15 g	
Calories 90	Sodium 710 mg	30%	Protein 2 g	
Fat calories 0	Vitamin A 12% · Vitamin C 12% · Calcium 0% · Iron 0%			

*Percent daily values (%DV) are based on a 2,000 calorie diet.

1. If $\frac{1}{2}$ cup of soup equals 120 milliliters, then how many milliliters (mL) are in $3\frac{1}{2}$ cups of soup?

2. If a can has 2.5 servings, how many cans are needed to serve 10 people?

3. One serving contains 90 calories, how many calories are in $4\frac{1}{2}$ servings?

4. One gram of fiber constitutes 4% of a daily dietary value. How many grams of fiber would be present in 25% of the daily value?

5. How many grams of carbohydrates are present if the portion meets 15% of the daily value of carbohydrates? Round to the nearest tenth.

Use the information from the label to complete these proportions.

Big Al's Organic Sweet and Juicy Dried Plums

Nutrition facts Serving size 1½ oz (40 g in about 5 dried plums) Servings per container about 30		Amount per serving Calories 100 Calories from fat 0	
	%DV*		%DV*
Total fat 0 g	0%	Potassium 290 mg	8%
Saturated fat 0 g	0%	Total carbohydrates 24 g	8%
Cholesterol 0 mg	0%	Dietary fiber 3 g	11%
Sodium 5 mg	0%	Soluble fiber 1 g	
Vitamin A 10% (100% as beta carotene)		Insoluble fiber 1 g	
Vitamin C 0%	·	Sugars 12 g	
Calcium 2%		Protein 1 g	
Iron 2%			
		Big Al's Organic Sweet and Juicy Dried Plums/Prunes	

*Percent daily values (%DV) are based on a 2,000 calorie diet. Your daily values may be higher or lower depending on your calorie needs.

6. How many total grams (g) of weight are present in 34 prunes?

7. If 100 calories are consumed with 5 prunes, how many calories are consumed with 12 prunes?

8. If 5 prunes have 290 milligrams (mg) of potassium and that accounts for 8% of percent daily value, how many prunes are needed to equal 15% of the percent daily value? Round to the nearest whole number.

9. If 5 prunes equals 10% of the Vitamin A needed daily, what percent of the daily % of Vitamin A is present in 20 prunes?

10. If a serving size is $1\frac{1}{2}$ ounces (oz), how many ounces are five servings?

Use the information from the label to complete these proportions.

Jade's Soy Milk

Nutrition facts	Amount/serving %DV*		Amount/serving %DV*	
Serving size 1 cup (240 ml)	Total fat 4 g	6%	Total Carbohydrates 4 g 1%	
Servings about 8 per 1.89 L	Saturated fat 0.5 g	3%	Fiber 1 g	4%
Calories 80	Trans fat 0 g		Cholesterol 0 mg	0%
Fat calories 35	Polyunsaturated fat 2.5 g		Sugars 12 g	
	Monounsaturated fat 1 g		Protein 7 g	
	Sodium 85 mg 4%		Potassium 300 mg	8%
	Vitamin A 10% · Vitamin C 0% · Calcium 30% · Iron 6%			
	Vitamin D 10% · Folate 6% · Magnesium 10% · Selenium 8%			

*Percent daily values (%DV) are based on a 2,000 calorie diet.

11. If 1 cup of soup contains 4 grams (g) total fat, then how many grams of total fat are in $2\frac{3}{4}$ cups of Jade's Soy Milk?

12. If a cup of soy milk contains 85 milligrams of sodium, and an individual consumes $2\frac{2}{3}$ cups of soy milk per day, what is the sodium intake from soy milk? Round to the nearest whole number.

13. If one serving of Jade's Soy Milk provides 1% of the daily carbohydrates. How many milliliters make 5% of the daily carbohydrate intake?

14. One serving contains 80 calories, how many calories are in $3\frac{1}{4}$ servings?

15. If 1 cup of Jade's Soy Milk provides 1 gram of fiber and 4% of the recommended daily fiber intake, how many cups of this soy milk are needed to make 25% of the dietary fiber?

RATIO AND PROPORTION SELF-TEST

Show all your work.

1. Write a definition for proportion. Provide one health profession application or example.

2. $30 : 120 = ? : 12$

3. 1 glass contains 8 ounces. How many full glasses are in 78 ounces?

4. $\frac{1}{2} : 4 = \frac{1}{3} : x$

5. $x : 625 = 1 : 5$

6. If 10 milligrams are contained in 2 milliliters, how many milligrams are contained in 28 milliliters?

7. A tablet contains 30 milligrams of medication. How many tablets will be needed to provide Ms Smith with 240 milligrams of medication?

8. 100 micrograms of a drug are contained in 2 cubic centimeters. How many cubic centimeters are contained in 15 micrograms?

9. $\dfrac{1}{100} : 6 = \ ? : 8$

10. $0.04 : 0.5 = 0.12 : \ ?$

11. How many minutes are in 130 seconds? Your answer will have both minutes and seconds. Show your setup.

12. Four out of every six dental patients request fluoride treatment after their dental cleaning treatments. If 120 patients have dental cleanings this week, how many will choose to have fluoride treatments as well?

13. If the doctor's office uses 128 disposal thermometer covers each day, how many covers will be used in a five-day workweek?

14. Solve: $\dfrac{1}{125} : 3 :: \underline{\hphantom{xxx}} : 12$

15. If the doctor ordered six ounces of cranberry juice four times a day for four days, how many total ounces would be served the patient?

Unit 5

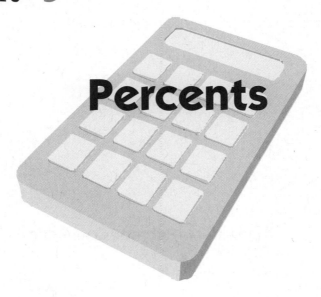

Percents

Percents are another example of a part-to-whole relationship in math. Percents are *parts of one hundred* and are represented by the % sign. Percents can be written as fractions: 35 parts of 100 or $^{35}/_{100}$.

Knowledge of percents in health care will help you understand the strength in percent of solutions for patient medications, interest on loans and taxes, and discounts and markups in pharmacies and retail stores. In general, percent applications are seen less frequently than fractions and decimals by general health care professionals.

Percent-to-Decimal Conversion

To convert a percent to a decimal, shift the decimal point two places to the *left*. The process of doing this quick division replaces having to divide the number by 100. This is the same method of simplified division as shown in Unit 3: Decimals.

> A whole number has its decimal to the far right of the final digit or number.
>
> $$125\% = 125.\% \qquad 76\% = 76.\%$$

Example

$$75\% \rightarrow 7\ 5.\% \rightarrow 0.75$$
$$\cup \cup$$

If a percent has a fractional part, the decimal occurs between the whole number and the fractional part.

Example
$$33\frac{1}{3}\% \rightarrow 33.\frac{1}{3}\% \rightarrow 0.33\frac{1}{3}$$

Practice   Convert from percents to decimals:

1. 45%

2. 57%

3. $78\frac{1}{5}\%$

4. 101%

5. $44\frac{1}{2}\%$

Decimal-to-Percent Conversion

To convert a decimal to a percent, shift the decimal point two places to the *right*. This is the simplified multiplication method as practiced in Unit 3: Decimals.

   If a number has a decimal in it and you are converting from a decimal to a percent, use the existing decimal point as the starting point for the conversion. It is possible to have percents greater than 100.

> Begin counting from wherever the decimal is placed.
>
> $$0.023 \rightarrow 02.3\% \quad 2.56 \rightarrow 256\%$$
>
> Handle a mixed fraction by placing the decimal point between whole number and the fraction, then convert the fraction to a whole number by dividing the numerator by the denominator. Then move the decimal two places right and add a % sign.
>
> $$14\frac{3}{4} \rightarrow 14.\frac{3}{4} \rightarrow 14.75 \rightarrow 1475\%$$
> $$\cup\,\cup$$

Examples
$$0.25 \rightarrow 0.2\,5\% = 25\%$$
$$\cup\,\cup$$

$$13 \rightarrow 13. \rightarrow 13.0\,0 = 1300\%$$
$$\cup\,\cup$$

Practice   Convert from decimals to percents:

1. 0.625

2. 55.75

3. 8.6

4. 12.5

5. 0.076

Mixed Practice
Convert

1. 76.89% to a decimal

2. 0.05% to a decimal

3. 86% to a decimal

4. 6.25 to a percent

5. 0.078 to a percent

6. $9\frac{3}{4}$ to a percent

7. $1.25\frac{1}{4}$ to a percent

8. $78\frac{1}{9}\%$ to a decimal

9. 1.5% to a decimal

10. $0.67\frac{1}{4}$ to a percent

Using Proportion to Solve Percent Problems

Proportions are also very useful in solving percent problems. To accomplish this, use the formula

$$\frac{\%}{100} = \frac{\text{is (the part)}}{\text{whole (the total)}}$$

To solve any percent problem, take the information from the problem and put it into the formula. There are three possible places that the information can go.

$$\frac{?}{100} = \frac{?}{?}$$

The 100 never changes because that indicates that every percent is part of 100. It is important to set up the problem correctly. The following questions ask for different information. Therefore, the setup of the problems will be different.

Problem	Setup
What is 25% of 75?	$\frac{25}{100} = \frac{?}{75}$
What % of 75 is 18.75?	$\frac{?}{100} = \frac{18.75}{75}$
18.75 is 25% of what?	$\frac{25}{100} = \frac{18.75}{?}$

Note that the ? is in a different place each time. When the problem is worked, each of the above answers will be different.

Practice   Set up the problems, but do not solve.

1. What is 25% of 200?

2. 75 is what % of 125?

3. Find 8.5% of 224.

4. 40 percent of what number is 350?

5. 18 is what percent of 150?

6. What is $1\frac{1}{2}$% of 400?

7. 75 of 90 is what percent?

8. Out of 200, 140 is what percent?

9. 50% of what number is 75?

10. $8\frac{1}{3}$% of 144 is what?

To solve percent problems in health care, one needs to be aware that the problem may include whole numbers, fractions, and decimals. The skills used in percents draw on the foundation you have in these areas of math computation. It is important to remember and apply the fraction concepts learned when dealing with fractions in percents because a fraction is more accurate and exact than a decimal number that has a repeating final digit.

   To solve percent problems, use the proportion method studied in Unit 4: Ratio and Proportion.

Example   Fifteen is what percent of 300?

$$\frac{x\%}{100} = \frac{15}{300}$$

Step 1: Cross multiply the two numbers.

$$(100 \times 15 = 1500)$$

Step 2: Divide the step 1 answer by the remaining number—the number diagonal from the x or ?

$$1{,}500 \div 300 = 5$$

The answer is 5%. So we know that 15 is 5% of 300.

Practice   1. 15% of 120 is _____.

2. 33 is what % of 44?

3. 62 is what percent of 248?

4. 40% of 120 is what?

5. What is 35% of 16.8?

6. Find 9% of 3,090.

7. 45 is what percent of 200?

8. 74 is what percent of 74?

9. What is 44% of 40?

10. 121 is what % of 220?

   More complex percents include fractions, and the most efficient way of handling these is as complex fractions. By setting up the problem in proportion format, the work is put into manageable steps. A common error is that students multiply the first two numbers and consider their work done; however, there is always a final division step that must be performed.

Example   What is $8\frac{1}{3}$% of 150?

$$\frac{8\frac{1}{3}}{100} = \frac{x}{150}$$

Step 1:   Multiply $8\frac{1}{3}$ and 150. Deal with the fraction; do not change it to a decimal because if you do, your answer will not be as exact. Convert the mixed fraction into an improper fraction. Multiply the whole number by the denominator and add the numerator. Place this number over the denominator. Then multiply this improper fraction by the number 150.

$$8\frac{1}{3} = \frac{25}{3} \times 150 = \frac{3,750}{3} = 1250$$

Step 2:   Divide the step 1 answer of 1,250 by 100. Use simplified division. Simplified division moves the decimal 2 places to the left to divide by 100.

$$1,250 : 1,2\,5\,0 = 12.5 \text{ or } 12\frac{1}{2} \quad 0.5 \text{ equals } \frac{1}{2}.$$
$$\underset{\cup\ \cup}{}$$

Practice

1. What is $33\frac{1}{3}$% of 125? Round to the nearest hundredth.

2. $1\frac{1}{2}$% of 400 is what?

3. $66\frac{2}{3}$% of 90 is what?

4. $35\frac{1}{4}$% is what part of 150? Round to the nearest hundredth.

5. $12\frac{1}{2}$% of 125 is what? Round to the nearest hundredth.

6. 50 is $83\frac{1}{3}$% of what number?

7. 160 is $12\frac{1}{2}$% of what number?

8. 45 is $15\frac{1}{3}$% of what number? Round to the nearest hundredth.

9. 200 is $37\frac{1}{2}$% of what number? Round to the nearest hundredth.

10. $87\frac{1}{2}$% of 120 is what?

Two other applications of percents are important for the health care student: the percent strength of a solution and the single trade discount.

Percent Strength of Solutions

The strength of solutions is an important application of percents. A solution is a liquid that has had medication, minerals, or other products dissolved in it. Percent strength refers to how much of a substance has been dissolved in a specific amount of liquid.

Key to percent strength is your knowledge of part-to-whole relationships: A percent is x parts to 100 total parts. Solution refers to a two-part substance: a solute that is the drug, mineral, or product and a solvent or liquid that can be a variety depending on the medical application. Solutes will occur either as a dry drug measured in grams or as a liquid measured in milliliters. The total volume of the liquid is always in milliliters.

Example   A 15% drug solution has 15 parts of drug to 100 parts of solution. There are 15 grams of drug to 100 milliliters of solution. As a ratio, this would be shown in the reduced form as 3 : 20.

Sometimes the solution will be given as a ratio rather than a percent. To express the solution strength as a percent, set up the problem as a proportion with 100 ml of the total solution. Recall that percent is always part of 100.

Practice   Percent strength: What is the ratio of pure drug to solution? Simplify, if necessary.

1. 4% solution   _____

2. 10% solution   _____

3. $1\frac{1}{2}$% solution   _____

4. 7.5% solution   _____

5. 5% solution   _____

Knowledge of proportion is useful in converting to smaller or larger amounts of solution. In health care, professionals may not always require 100 mL of a solution. It is important to maintain the correct ratio of pure drug to solution to ensure that the patient is getting the medication or solution the doctor intended. Note that the ratio of pure drug remains consistent no matter how much solution is to be prepared.

Example   Percent strength 8% means that there are 8 g of drug to 100 mL of solution. If the doctor orders 25 mL of an 8% strength solution, then a proportion may be used to ensure that the ratio of pure drug to solution represents 8%.

$$\frac{\overset{known}{8\text{ g of drugs}}}{100\text{ mL solution}} = \frac{\overset{unknown}{?\text{ g of drug}}}{25\text{ mL solution}}$$

Step 1: $8 \times 25 = 200$

Step 2: $200 \div 100 = 2$

So to make 25 mL of an 8% solution using this ratio of pure drug to solution, 2 g of pure drug to 25 mL of solution are required. This keeps the percent strength of the medication consistent with the doctor's order for an 8% strength solution. Note that the amount of mixed solution changes, not the percent strength itself.

Example   Ten grams of drug in 25 mL of solution. What is the percent strength of this medication?

To convert this ratio into a percent, write it as a proportion. Then solve for x which will become the percent.

$$\underset{\text{25 mL}}{\overset{\text{10 g}}{}} = \frac{x \text{ g}}{100 \text{ mL}}$$

$$\frac{\overset{known}{10 \text{ g}}}{25 \text{ mL}} = \frac{\overset{unknown}{x \text{ g}}}{100 \text{ mL}}$$

Follow proportion steps to solve. Cross multiply $10 \times 100 = 1000$. Divide 1000 by 25 = 40, so the answer is 40% strength.

Practice   1. The doctor has ordered a 5% saline solution to be prepared. How many grams of pure drug will be needed to make each of these amounts of solution at the 5% strength?

a. 25 mL of solution

b. 35 mL of solution

c. 65 mL of solution

d. 125 mL of solution

2. Nine milliliters of pure drug are in 100 mL of solution.

a. What is the percent strength of the solution?

b. How many milliliters of drug are in 75 mL of that solution?

3. Fifteen grams of pure drug are in 50 mL.

   a. What is the percent strength of the solution?

   b. How many grams of pure drug are in 200 mL of the solution?

Additional Practice with Solution Strength

1. A $12\frac{3}{4}$% strength solution has been prepared.

   a. How many grams of medication is in the $12\frac{3}{4}$% strength solution?

   b. How many milliliters of solution are in this $12\frac{3}{4}$% strength solution?

   c. Express this solution as a simplified ratio.

   d. How much pure drug is needed to create 35.5 mL of this solution? Round to the nearest tenth. Your answer will be in grams.

   e. How much pure drug is needed to create 80 mL of this solution? Your answer will be in grams.

   f. If you have 60 mL of solution, how many grams of pure drug will you have in order to keep the $12\frac{3}{4}$%? Round to the nearest tenth. Your answer will be in grams.

2. A 0.09% strength solution has been prepared.

   a. How many grams of medication is in the 0.09% strength solution?

   b. How many milliliters of solution are in this 0.09% strength solution?

   c. Express this solution as a simplified ratio.

   d. How much pure drug is needed to create 54 mL of this solution? Round to the nearest hundredth. Your answer will be in grams.

   e. How much pure drug is needed to create 24 mL of this solution? Round to the nearest hundredth. Your answer will be in grams.

   f. If you have 50 mL of solution, how many grams of pure drug will you have in order to keep the 0.09% solution. Round to the nearest hundredth. Your answer will be in grams.

3. A 78% strength solution has been prepared.

   a. How many grams of medication is in the 78% strength solution?

   b. How many milliliters of solution are in this 78% strength solution?

   c. Express this solution as a simplified ratio.

   d. How much pure drug is needed to create 65.5 mL of this solution? Round to the nearest tenth. Your answer will be in grams.

   e. How much pure drug is needed to create 90 mL of this solution? Round to the nearest tenth. Your answer will be in grams.

   f. If you have 450 mL of solution, how many grams of pure drug will you have in order to keep the 78%? Your answer will be in grams.

Single Trade Discount

Single trade discounts are useful to individuals who handle products or inventory that must be marked up. The single trade discount provides the net price of items when a single discount has been given. Some health care organizations that use certain name brands receive these discounts from manufacturers of the products they use or sell most often.

Example   What is the net price of a surgical instrument listed at $189.90 with a trade discount of 40%?

Step 1: The percentage is first made into a decimal by moving the decimal point two places to the left. Then, multiply the list price by the trade discount.

> You may need to round your decimal number to the nearest cent.

$$\begin{array}{r} \$189.90 \\ \times\ \ .40 \\ \hline 00000 \\ 75960 \\ \hline \$75.96 \end{array}$$

Step 2: Subtract the amount of the discount (the answer from step 1) from the list price to get the net price.

$$\begin{array}{r} \$189.90 \\ -75.96 \\ \hline \$113.94 \end{array}$$

The net price of this instrument is $113.94.

Practice Find the net price by using the single trade discount method. If necessary, round to the nearest penny. Show your work.

	List price	Trade discount	Amount of discount	Net price
1.	$475.50	15%	_____	_____
2.	$179.85	20%	_____	_____
3.	$125.55	12.5%	_____	_____
4.	$455.86	30%	_____	_____
5.	$352.90	25%	_____	_____
6.	$72.35	10%	_____	_____
7.	$250.40	45%	_____	_____
8.	$862.75	35%	_____	_____
9.	$158.00	40%	_____	_____
10.	$73.85	10%	_____	_____

PERCENT SELF-TEST

1. Write the definition of a percent. Provide one example.

2. Convert the following into percents:

   a. $0.87\frac{1}{4}$

   b. $\frac{5}{6}$

3. 75% of 325 is what number?

4. 8 is what % of 40?

5. 28 is 14% of what number?

6. What does $5\frac{1}{2}$% solution mean?

7. The doctor has ordered 25 mL of 9% saline solution. How much pure drug is needed to make this order?

8. The list price for a case of medicine is $129.50. Your pharmacy will receive a 12% trade discount.

   a. What is the amount of the discount? _____

   b. What is the net cost of a case of medicine? _____

9. What percent is 3 tablets of a prescription written for 36 tablets?

10. If a pharmacy gave a 15% discount on walkers, what would be the discount for a total bill of $326.00 for a six-month rental?

11. If a ratio of 3 : 25 is given for a solution, what percent strength is this solution?

12. What is $\frac{1}{2}$% of 500?

13. Express 8 : 125 as a percent.

14. What is $\frac{3}{4}$% of 20?

15. 35 is 0.05% of what?

Unit 6

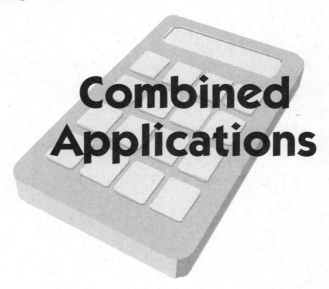

Combined Applications

Health care workers rely on a variety of math systems to achieve their daily tasks. Knowledge of ways to convert efficiently between systems will benefit you on the job as your expertise grows and your circle of responsibility increases. It is important to have the ability to convert between fractions, decimals, ratios, and percents. Although these skills have been separately reviewed, they are brought together here to develop some strategies for doing these conversions in the most efficient way.

Conversions among Fractions, Decimals, Ratios, and Percent

Review the basics of conversion:

Conversion	Method/Formula
Fraction to decimal	Divide the denominator into the numerator.

$$\frac{3}{4} = \begin{array}{r} 0.75 \\ 4\overline{)3.0} \\ \underline{28}\downarrow \\ 20 \\ \underline{20} \\ 0 \end{array}$$

Decimal to fraction	Count the decimal places, place the number over 1 with zeros to match the same number of decimal places.

$$0.0\underline{2} \text{ (2 places)} \rightarrow \frac{2}{10\underline{0}} \text{ (2 zeros)}$$

Reduce to $^1/_{50}$.

Proper fraction to ratio, ratio to proper fraction	Ratios are shown with : instead of /. Fractions and ratios are interchangeable simply by changing the symbol.

$$\frac{1}{8} \rightarrow 1:8 \text{ and } 4:31 \rightarrow \frac{4}{31}$$

The first ratio number is always the numerator and the second ratio number is always the denominator. All fractions and ratios must be in lowest terms.

Mixed number to ratio, ratio to mixed number	If the fraction is a mixed number, the mixed number first must be made into an improper fraction before setting up the ratio.

$$1\frac{3}{4} \rightarrow 1 \times 4 + 3 = \frac{7}{4} \rightarrow 7:4$$

If the ratio is an improper fraction when the conversion is made, make it a mixed number.

$$\frac{11}{4} \rightarrow 11 \div 4 = 2\frac{3}{4}$$

Decimal to percent	Move the decimal point two places to the right. Add the percent sign.

$$0.25 \rightarrow 25\% \quad 1.456 \rightarrow 145.6\%$$

Percent to decimal	Move the decimal point two places to the left. Add zeros if needed as placeholders.

$$90\% \rightarrow 0.9 \text{ and } 5\% \rightarrow 0.05$$

$$57\frac{1}{2}\% \rightarrow 0.57\frac{1}{2} \text{ or } 0.575$$

Fraction to percent	Convert fraction to decimal, then to percent.
Decimal to ratio	Convert decimal to fraction, then change sign to ratio.

Convert the following numbers to the other number systems. Using the review sheet of conversion methods, try to compute only one math problem per line by carefully selecting the order of the conversions to be done. By carefully selecting the order of conversions, you will minimize extra work.

Example

Fraction	Decimal	Ratio	Percent
_____	0.05	_____	_____

Figuring out the order takes a little practice. When 0.05 is changed to a percent first, no math calculation needs to be done: Simply move the decimal.

Fraction	Decimal	Ratio	Percent
_____	0.05	_____	5%

Next convert the decimal to a fraction. Count the number of decimal places and then place the 5 over a 1 with the same number of zeros as the decimal places. Reduce the fraction to lowest terms.

Fraction	Decimal	Ratio	Percent
$\frac{5}{100} \rightarrow \frac{1}{20}$	0.05	_____	5%

Take the reduced fraction and write it in ratio form.

Fraction	Decimal	Ratio	Percent
$\frac{5}{100} \rightarrow \frac{1}{20}$	0.05	$1:20$	5%

Example

Fraction	Decimal	Ratio	Percent
$7\frac{3}{5}$	_____	_____	_____

This mixed number must be made into an improper fraction before it can become a ratio.

$$\left(7 \times 5 + 3 = 38 \rightarrow \frac{38}{5} \right)$$

Change the signs from / to : to make the ratio.

Fraction	Decimal	Ratio	Percent
$7\frac{3}{5}$	_____	$38:5$	_____

Next change to a decimal. Handle the whole number 7 separately. Place it on the line as a whole number, then divide the denominator into the numerator.

$$3 \div 5 = 0.6$$

Add this to the whole number to make 7.6.

Fraction	Decimal	Ratio	Percent
$7\frac{3}{5}$	7.6	38 : 5	_____

Finally, move the decimal point from the decimal number two places to the right. Add the percent sign.

Fraction	Decimal	Ratio	Percent
$7\frac{3}{5}$	7.6	38 : 5	760%

Suggested Order of Operations

If starting with percent, move from → decimal → fraction → ratio.

If starting with ratio, move from → fraction → decimal → percent.

If starting with fraction, move from → ratio → decimal → percent.

If starting with decimal, move from → percent → fraction → ratio.

Some conversions can be memorized easily:

$$\frac{1}{2} \to 0.5 \to 50\%$$

$$\frac{1}{4} \to 0.25 \to 25\%$$

$$\frac{3}{4} \to 0.75 \to 75\%$$

$$\frac{1}{3} \to 0.33\frac{1}{3} \to 33\frac{1}{3}\%$$

$$\frac{2}{3} \to 0.66\frac{2}{3} \to 66\frac{2}{3}\%$$

Provide the following measures. Reduce to lowest terms as necessary. Round to the nearest hundredth, if necessary.

	Fraction	Decimal	Ratio	Percent
1.	$\frac{3}{4}$	_____	_____	_____
2.	_____	_____	1 : 20	_____

	Fraction	Decimal	Ratio	Percent
3.	_____	_____	_____	50%
4.	_____	0.625	_____	_____
5.	_____	_____	1 : 250	_____
6.	$\frac{7}{8}$	_____	_____	_____
7.	_____	0.06	_____	_____
8.	_____	_____	_____	12.5%
9.	$\frac{1}{10}$	_____	_____	_____
10.	_____	_____	_____	$33\frac{1}{3}\%$
11.	_____	1.36	_____	_____
12.	$12\frac{1}{2}$	_____	_____	_____
13.	_____	_____	2 : 5	_____
14.	_____	$0.66\frac{2}{3}$	_____	_____
15.	_____	_____	16 : 25	_____
16.	_____	0.004	_____	_____
17.	$\frac{5}{6}$	_____	_____	_____
18.	_____	_____	_____	$7\frac{1}{4}\%$
19.	_____	0.01	_____	_____
20.	_____	_____	7 : 3	_____

Using Combined Applications in Measurement Conversion

In health care, a solid working knowledge of weights and measures is essential. Three systems of measure will be used in your work: household or standard measurement, metric measurement, covered in this unit, and apothecary measurement, covered in Unit 11: Dosage Calculations. Critical to your success in measurement conversion is your ability to remember a few key conversions and the proportion method for solving conversions. Metric-to-metric conversions use a different conversion method, which is also covered in Unit 11.

Household or standard measurements are used by all of us in our daily activities. Household measures tend to be less accurate than either metric or apothecary measures because of their nature and our methods of using them. So household measures are used in the less critical measurements in health care. Abbreviations of units of measure are used and some new abbreviations are introduced below:

Drop = gtt

Teaspoon = t (tsp)

Tablespoon = T (tbsp)

Practice   Write the word for each abbreviation.

1. ft. = _____   6. t = _____

2. yd. = _____   7. qt. = _____

3. oz. = _____   8. pt. = _____

4. T = _____   9. gtt = _____

5. lb. = _____   10. gal. = _____

Standard Units of Measure

The basics of standard measure conversion were covered in Unit 4: Ratio and Proportion. To refresh yourself on the application of proportion to measurement conversions, complete the review exercises.

Time
1 minute = 60 seconds
1 day   = 24 hours
1 week   = 7 days
1 year   = 12 months

Weight
1 kilogram = 2.2 pounds
1 pound   = 16 ounces

Linear Measure
1 foot   = 12 inches
1 yard   = 3 feet
1 meter = 39.4 inches
1 inch   = 2.5 or 2.54 centimeters

Liquid Measure
1 tablespoon = 3 teaspoons
1 cup   = 8 ounces
1 pint   = 2 cups
1 quart   = 2 pints
1 gallon   = 4 quarts

Approximate Equivalents
grain i   = 60 milligrams
1 teaspoon   = 5 milliliters
1 tablespoon   = 3 teaspoons
fluid dram 1   = 4 milliliters
fluid ounce 1 = fluid drams 8
fluid ounce 1 = 2 tablespoons
fluid ounce 1 = 30 milliliters
1 cup   = 250 milliliters
               = fluid ounces 8
1 pint   = 500 milliliters
               = 2 cups or fluid ounces 16
1 quart   = fluid ounces 32
               = 1 liter or 1000 milliliters
1 cubic centimeter = 1 milliliter
1 kilogram   = 2.2 pounds
fluid ounce 1 = 2 tablespoons

Review   Use the provided tables to assist you in proportion conversions.

1. 1250 milliliters = _____ pints

2. 15 kilograms = _____ pounds

3. 12.5 inches = _____ centimeters

4. _____ milliliters = 13 teaspoons

5. _____ ounces = 90 milliliters

6. 38.1 centimeters = _____ inches

7. _____ ounces = $1\frac{1}{2}$ pints

8. _____ quarts = 15 liters

9. _____ teaspoons = 12.5 milliliters

10. _____ cubic centimeters = 15 teaspoons

More Combined Applications

Sometimes measurement conversions require more than one conversion to get to the answer.

Example   Two conversions are required to convert from ounces to teaspoons.

Step 1: Convert the ounces to milliliters:

$$\underset{\text{known}}{\frac{1 \text{ ounce}}{20 \text{ mL}}} = \underset{\text{unknown}}{\frac{8 \text{ ounces}}{? \text{ mL}}} \rightarrow 160 \text{ milliliters}$$

Step 2: Convert milliliters to teaspoons.

$$\frac{1 \text{ teaspoon}}{5 \text{ mL}} = \frac{? \text{ teaspoons}}{160 \text{ mL}} \rightarrow 32 \text{ teaspoons}$$

These problems cannot be solved by making a straight conversion from what is known to what is unknown. A path must be developed so that you can establish how to get the answer. Think about what conversions most closely match the problem itself, then set up the problem.

> Do not rush through the two-step conversions. These require some forethought about how to get from what is known to what is unknown.

Plastic medicine cups are used in the health care industry to measure liquid dosages. A medicine cup is typically marked off in milliliters. Often one medicine cup is 1 fluid ounce, which is 30 mL.

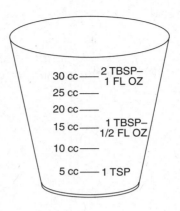

Practice   1. 1 medicine cup = _____ teaspoons

2. 3 teaspoons = _____ (drops)

3. $2\frac{1}{4}$ pints = _____ ounces

4. 1 cup = _____ teaspoons

5. 1 pint = _____ tablespoons

6. 15 tablespoons = _____ cubic centimeters

7. 68,000 grams = _____ pounds

8. 28 inches = _____ millimeters

9. _____ ounces = 24 teaspoons

10. $1\frac{1}{2}$ ounces = _____ teaspoons

Sometimes math problems require multiple setups. To solve these, group the work into the most logical format.

Example $$\frac{25\%}{\frac{1}{4}}$$

Step 1: Look at the problem and decide what to do to make the units similar. Convert 25% into a fraction.

$$\rightarrow \frac{25}{100}$$

Step 2: Review the problem to see what operation should be completed.

$$\frac{\frac{25}{100}}{\frac{1}{4}}$$

This problem is a complex fraction. Divide the denominator of $\frac{1}{4}$ into the numerator of $\frac{25}{100}$.

$$\frac{25}{100} \div \frac{1}{4} \rightarrow \frac{25}{100} \times \frac{4}{1} = \frac{100}{100} = 1$$

**Mixed Review
Practice**

1. $\dfrac{50\%}{\frac{1}{4}}$

2. $\dfrac{1:150}{1:300} \times 2$

3. $12\frac{1}{2}\% \times \dfrac{\frac{1}{2}}{\frac{3}{4}}$

4. $\dfrac{\frac{1}{2}\%}{4} \times 1000$

5. $5\% \times \dfrac{1:2}{3:4}$

**Converting among
Systems
Worksheet**

Provide the following measures. Reduce to lowest terms as necessary.

	Fraction	Decimal	Ratio	Percent
1.	$\frac{7}{8}$	_____	_____	_____
2.	_____	_____	1 : 30	_____
3.	_____	_____	_____	75%
4.	$\frac{1}{17}$	_____	_____	_____
5.	_____	_____	2 : 5	_____
6.	$\frac{5}{6}$	_____	_____	_____
7.	_____	0.08	_____	_____
8.	_____	_____	_____	10.25%

	Fraction	Decimal	Ratio	Percent
9.	$\frac{3}{5}$	_____	_____	_____
10.	_____	_____	1 : 200	_____
11.	_____	1.625	_____	_____
12.	$\frac{1}{8}$	_____	_____	_____
13.	_____	_____	11 : 50	_____
14.	_____	0.15	_____	_____
15.	_____	_____	3 : 25	_____
16.	_____	0.008	_____	_____
17.	$\frac{1}{6}$	_____	_____	_____
18.	_____	_____	_____	$15\frac{1}{4}\%$
19.	_____	0.04	_____	_____
20.	_____	_____	9 : 10,000	_____

COMBINED APPLICATIONS SELF-TEST

Show all your work.

1. Convert $\frac{3}{75}$ to a decimal.

2. Convert $\frac{1}{2}\%$ to a ratio.

3. Convert 1.05 to a fraction.

4. Convert $4\frac{1}{8}$ to a ratio.

5. Convert $27\frac{1}{4}$ to a decimal.

6. Convert 12 : 200 to a percent.

7. Convert 14.25% to a ratio.

8. $3\frac{1}{4}$ cups = _____ ounces

9. 12 fluid ounces = _____ tablespoons

10. $3\frac{1}{2}$ feet = _____ centimeters

11. 18 hours = _____ minutes

12. 1 gallon = _____ cups

13. If a teaspoon has approximately 60 drops, how many drops are in $2\frac{1}{3}$ tablespoons?

14. $12\% \times 0.67$

15. $\dfrac{15\%}{\frac{1}{2}}$

Unit 7

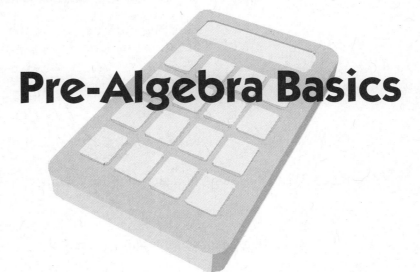

Pre-Algebra Basics

Algebra is the study, understanding, and use of symbolic reasoning, mathematical properties, processes, and calculations to problem solve for a variety of unknown situations. This unit lays the foundation for algebraic concepts that you may need later in your training.

Integers

We use integers to solve many everyday math problems. The integers consist of the positive whole numbers (1, 2, 3, 4, 5, . . .), their negatives (-1, -2, -3, -4, -5, . . .), and the number zero. Zero is neither positive or negative; it is neutral. Integers form a countable infinite set.

The number line is a line labeled with the integers in increasing order from left to right. The number line extends in both directions:

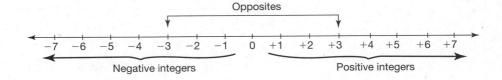

The ($-$) sign is used to show a negative number and the ($+$) sign is used to show a positive number.

Remember that any integer on the right is always greater than the integer on the left.

135

We can use the + and − sign to illustrate numbers for information. For example, if the hospital adds three more staff, that can be illustrated as +3. Use the chart to help decide if the number is negative or positive.

Terms that indicate a negative integer	Terms that indicate a positive integer
decrease	increase
less	more
loss	profit
fewer	more

Practice   Write the integer for each of the following situations:

1. 25 more nurses _____

2. a 1 degree increase in temperature _____

3. a profit of two thousand dollars _____

4. a twelve pound loss in weight _____

5. 12 beats a minute less _____

Write the opposite of each integer:

1. −34 _____

2. 12 _____

3. +5 _____

4. −100 _____

5. +17 _____

Provide two examples when positive or negative integers might be used to represent a health care situation.

1. _____

2. _____

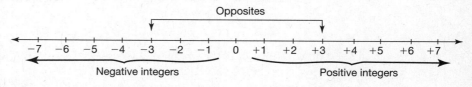

We can use the symbols of <, >, and = to represent the number relationships.

For example,

$$-8 > -12 \quad \text{(Remember that the negative numbers increase}$$
$$-4 < 2 \qquad \text{in value closer to zero)}$$
$$12 > -6$$
$$-3 = -3$$

Practice   Compare the following with $<$, $>$, or $=$

1. $+6$ _____ -34

2. -4 _____ -2

3. $+12$ _____ -16

4. -8 _____ -8

5. -24 _____ $+24$

Absolute Value

The absolute value of an integer tells its distance from zero on the number line. The absolute value of a number such as 3, is shown as | 3 |. The straight bars indicate the distance of a number from zero. This is why absolute value is never negative; absolute value only asks "how far?", whether the number is in a positive or negative direction on the number line. This means that | 3 | = 3 because 3 is three units to the right of zero, and also | −3 | = 3, because −3 is three units to the left of zero. So whether it is | 3 | or | −3 |, the distance from zero in both cases is 3.
For example,

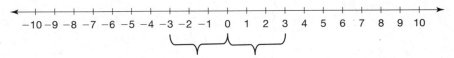

The absolute value of | +7 | = 7.

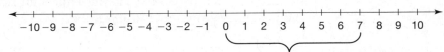

The absolute value of | −5 | = 5.

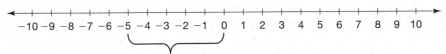

The absolute value of | 4 | = 4.

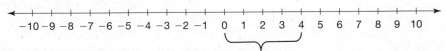

Practice   Write the absolute value of the following:

1. $| +4 |$ = _____

2. $| -14 |$ = _____

3. $| 6 |$ = _____

4. $| 21 |$ = _____

5. $| -476 |$ = _____

Integer Operations

Integer operations use the basic mathematical functions as addition, subtraction, multiplication, and division to solve math problems.

Adding Integers with the Same Sign

To add positive integers is just like adding whole numbers. For example, $2 + 7 = 9$ is the same as $+2 + +7 = +9$. Thus, the numbers move right on the number line.

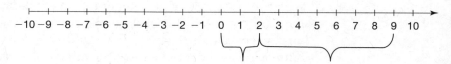

To add negative integers, the movement along the number line will be to the left of 0.

So $-4 + -3 = -7$. Thus, when two negative numbers are added, the sum will be a larger negative number.

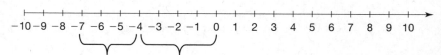

Remember that the absolute value is the distance from zero on the number line. So to add integers having the same sign, add their absolute values and then use the same sign as the numbers you are adding.

Examples

$5 + 4 =$ _____	$-7 + 0 =$ _____	$-7 + -5 =$ _____
The absolute values are $|5| + |4| = 9$ These are positive numbers being added.	The absolute values are $|7| + |0| = 7$ Adding zero to any number does not change the number. Add the negative sign.	The absolute values are $|7| + |5| = 12$ Add the sign of the numbers being added.
$5 + 4 = 9$	$-7 + 0 = -7$	$-7 + -5 = -12$

Practice

1. $4 + 7 =$

2. $-9 + -7 =$

3. $-8 + 0 =$

4. $23 + 12 =$

5. $-12 + -54 =$

6. $(-5) + -18 =$

7. $3 + 6 + 12 =$

8. $(-9) + (-5) + (-12) =$

9. $(-17) + (-2) + (-3) =$

10. $(2) + 0 + (14) =$

Adding Integers with Different Signs

The number line is very helpful in adding numbers with different signs. The number line below shows the sum of $-5 + 8$.

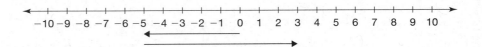

The integer -5 plus 8 equals 3. Note that the positive 8 is larger than the negative 5, so the answer will be $+3$ or 3.

Remember that the absolute value is the distance from zero on the number line. So to add integers having the different signs, subtract their absolute values and then use the sign of the larger number.

Examples

$-7 + 6 =$ _____	$+9 + (-4) =$ _____	$(-8) + (-5) + 7 =$ _____
Subtract the absolute values. $\lvert 7 \rvert - \lvert 6 \rvert = 1$ The -7 is larger than the 6. The answer will be negative.	Subtract the absolute values $\lvert 9 \rvert - \lvert 4 \rvert = 5$ The $+9$ is larger than -4. The answer will be positive.	Combine the integers with the same signs. $(-8) + (-5) = -13$ Subtract the absolute values $\lvert 13 \rvert - \lvert 7 \rvert = 6$ The -13 is larger than the 7. The answer will be negative.
$-7 + 6 = -1$	$+9 + (-4) = 5$	$(-8) + (-5) + 7 = -6$

Practice

1. $12 + (-7) =$

2. $-9 + 11 =$

3. $23 + -8 =$

4. $-7 + 13 =$

5. $8 + (-12) + 10 =$

6. $-3 + 4 + (-7) =$

7. $6 + (-5) + (-11) =$

8. $-28 + 45 + (+12) =$

9. $98 + (-12) + (-2) =$

10. $-7 + (0) + (-2) =$

Subtracting Integers

Each integer has an opposite. For example, $+5$ has an opposite integer, -5. This concept of opposites is used in the subtraction of integers. To subtract an integer, add its opposite. Addition and subtraction are inverse or opposite operations.

    Another way to explain how to subtract integers is to follow a three-step set up.

Look at the math problem: $+5 - (-9) = \underline{\hphantom{xxx}}$

Step 1: Change the math function sign from $-$ to $+$ $+5 + (-9) = \underline{\hphantom{xxx}}$

Step 2: Change the number sign after the $+5 + (+9) = \underline{\hphantom{xxx}}$
           function sign

Step 3: Add to find the solution $+5 - (-9) = 14$

If this looks confusing, count the spaces on the number line to discover the absolute value of each integer from 0.

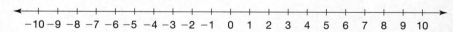

Examples

$8 - (-3) = \underline{\hphantom{xxx}}$	$-9 - 4 = \underline{\hphantom{xxx}}$	$-12 - (-5) = \underline{\hphantom{xxx}}$
Change the minus sign to add	Change the minus sign to add	Change the minus sign to add
$8 + (-3) = \underline{\hphantom{xxx}}$	$-9 + 4 = \underline{\hphantom{xxx}}$	$-12 + (-5) = \underline{\hphantom{xxx}}$
Change to the opposite sign of (-3) which is $(+3)$	Change to the opposite sign of (4) which is (-4)	Change to the opposite sign of (-5) which is $(+5)$
Add	Add	Add
$8 + (+3) = 11$	$-9 + -4 = -13$	$-12 + (+5) = -7$

Practice   1. $12 - (-7) =$

2. $-9 - 11 =$

3. $-12 - (-8) =$

4. $-7 - (+13) =$

5. $8 - (-12) =$

6. $-3 - (-4) =$

7. $6 - (-5) - (-11) =$

8. $-18 - (-25) - (+12) =$

9. $-12 - 12 =$

10. $-7 - (0) - (-1) =$

Multiplication of Integers

The multiplication of integers can be presented in a variety of ways. In whole numbers, we saw multiplication problems that looked like this: $2 \times 4 = 8$.

In integers, multiplication presents itself in a variety of formats. The multiplication sign $\times$ is not used because it can easily become confused with a variable. *A variable is an unknown number.*

The important part of multiplication of integers has to do with determining if the product of the factors is positive or negative. Follow these rules:

Problem	Workspace	Explanation of sign
$+2(+3)$ or $2(3)$	$2 \times 3 = 6$	The product of two positive factors is positive.
$-7(-6)$	$7(6) = 42$	The product of two negative factors is positive.
$-5(+6)$	$-5(6) = -30$	The product of a negative factor and a positive factor is negative.

Examples

$+7(12) =$ _____ $-8(-3) =$ _____ $-3(125) =$ _____
   $7 \cdot 12 =$ _____ $8 \cdot 3 =$ _____ $3 \cdot 125 =$ _____

Two positive   Two negative factors   One positive factor
factors means   means the product   times one negative
the product   will be positive.   factor means the
will be positive.   product will be negative.

$7 \cdot 12 = +84$ or 84 $-8(-3) = +24$ or 24 $-3(125) = -375$

Practice   1. $-9(4) =$

2. $7(2) =$

3. $-8 \cdot 16 =$

4. $3(-15) =$

5. $-5(23) \cdot 2 =$

6. $2(-9)(-3) =$

7. $-5(-2)(-4) =$

8. $9(2)\left(\dfrac{1}{2}\right) =$

9. $3(2)(-4) =$

10. $-1(2)(-4) =$

Division of Integers

The division symbol is usually not used in algebra. A fraction bar is used to show division.

$$\frac{28}{(7)} \quad \text{or} \quad \frac{128}{-4}$$

Problem	Workspace	Explanation of sign
$+108 \div +3 = \underline{\hspace{1cm}}$	$+108 \div +3 = +36$ or 36	The product of two positive factors is positive.
$\dfrac{-51}{-3} = \underline{\hspace{1cm}}$	$\dfrac{-51}{-3} = +17$ or 17	The product of two negative factors is positive.
$\dfrac{-63}{3} = \underline{\hspace{1cm}}$	$\dfrac{-63}{3} = -21$	The product of a negative factor and a positive factor is negative.

Examples

$$\frac{+150}{(+3)} = \underline{\hspace{1cm}} \qquad \frac{-18}{(-3)} = \underline{\hspace{1cm}} \qquad \frac{125}{-5} = \underline{\hspace{1cm}}$$

$$+150 \div (+3) = \underline{\hspace{1cm}} \qquad -18 \div (-3) = \underline{\hspace{1cm}} \qquad 125 \div (-5) = \underline{\hspace{1cm}}$$

If the signs of both the divisor and the dividend are positive, then the quotient will be positive.

If the signs of both the divisor and the dividend are negative, then the quotient will be positive.

If the sign of the divisor or the dividend is negative and the other is positive, the quotient will be negative.

$$\frac{+150}{(+3)} = +50 \text{ or } 50 \qquad \frac{-18}{(-3)} = +6 \text{ or } 6 \qquad \frac{125}{-5} = -25$$

Practice

1. $\dfrac{+300}{25} =$

2. $\dfrac{63}{-9} =$

3. $\dfrac{+164}{-2} =$

4. $\dfrac{-14}{-2} =$

5. $\dfrac{-90}{15} =$

6. $\dfrac{-300}{-4} =$

7. $\dfrac{12.6}{-3} =$

8. $\dfrac{-1000}{-5} =$

9. $\dfrac{-24}{4} =$

10. $\dfrac{180}{-10} =$

Exponential Notation

Exponential notation is a useful means for writing a product of many factors. The base is the number being multiplied and the exponent is the number of times that the base is multiplied.

For example, $3 \cdot 3 \cdot 3 \cdot 3 \cdot 3$ becomes 3^5. The number 3 is the base and 5 is the exponent. The exponent tells us how many times the base is used as a factor. This number, 3^5, is read 3 to the fifth power.

So this example has three forms.

Exponential form (exponential notation)	3^5
Factor form (repeated multiplication)	$3 \cdot 3 \cdot 3 \cdot 3 \cdot 3$
Standard form	243

Some simple rules make using exponents easy.

Rule 1: Any number raised to the first power is always equal to itself. $7^1 = 7$

Any number without an exponent always has an exponent of 1 understood.

Rule 2: If a number is raised to the second power, we say it is *squared*. 5^2 is read as 5 squared.

Rule 3: If a number is raised to the third power, we say it is *cubed*. 4^3 is read as 4 cubed.

Rule 4: Any number (except 0) raised to the zero power is equal to 1.

$9^0 = 1$ and $121^0 = 1$ However, note that $0^4 = 0 \times 0 \times 0 \times 0 = 0$

Practice   Complete the chart:

	Exponential notation	Factor form/repeated multiplication	Standard form
1	8^3	_____	_____
2	_____	$10 \cdot 10 \cdot 10 \cdot 10$	_____
3	_____	_____	16
4	_____	$2 \cdot 2 \cdot 2 \cdot 2 \cdot 2 \cdot 2$	_____
5	7^2	_____	_____
6	_____	_____	144
7	5^0	_____	_____
8	_____	$15 \cdot 15$	_____
9	_____	_____	1
10	_____	$10 \cdot 10$	_____

Scientific Notation

Like exponential notation, scientific notation is an easy way to write very large or very small numbers. In scientific notation, a number is written as two factors in a product. The first factor is a digit between 0 and 10. The second factor is a power of 10.
For example,

$$5.14 \times 10^2$$

The first factor is a digit between 0 and 10. The second factor is a power of 10.

To write a number in scientific notation

Step 1: Move the decimal after the first digit between 0 and 10.

5   1   4   becomes   5.14

2 moves

In the number 514, the first factor is 5.14.

The exponent is the number of places you moved the decimal point.
In the number 514, you moved two places, so the exponent is 2. The exponent is positive because you have to move the decimal point to the right to get back to the original number.

Step 2: Finally, include your power of 10 and exponent when you write your product.

$$5.14 \times 10^2$$

Example

$$8.3 \times 10^{-3}$$

Step 1:   0.0 0 8 3 becomes 8.3

3 moves

In 0.0083, the first factor is 8.3

In the number 0.0083, you moved three places, so the exponent is 3. This exponent is negative since you must move the decimal point to the left to get back to the original number.

Step 2: Finally, include your power of 10 and exponent when you write your product.

$$8.3 \times 10^{-3}$$

Practice 1 Write each number in scientific notation.

1. $6,000 =$ _____

2. $50,400 =$ _____

3. $8,000,000 =$ _____

4. $0.901 =$ _____

5. $0.0722 =$ _____

6. $0.0000135 =$ _____

To change a number in scientific notation to standard form

As stated, the exponent on the power of 10 factor determines how many places to move the decimal point when changing from scientific notation to standard notation.

Step 1: If your exponent is positive, move the decimal point to the right.

Step 2: If your exponent is negative, move the decimal point to the left.

Positive exponents
Example: $9.2 \times 10^7 = 92,000,000$
Process: Move the decimal point seven places to the right

Negative exponents
Example: $7.6 \times 10^{-4} = 0.00076$
Process: Move the decimal point four places to the left

Scientific notation	Process	Number in standard form
6.4×10^3	Move decimal 3 places right	6,400
3.2×10^4	Move decimal 4 places right	32,000
7×10^7	Move decimal 7 places right	70,000,000
4×10^{-2}	Move decimal 2 places left	0.04
25×10^{-3}	Move decimal 3 places left	25×10^{-3}
1.8×10^{-5}	Move decimal 5 places left	0.000018

Practice Write each number in standard form.

1. $1.03 \times 10^4 =$ _____

2. $8.75 \times 10^6 =$ _____

3. $9 \times 10^7 =$ _____

4. $4.51 \times 10^{-2} =$ _____

5. $6.6 \times 10^{-5} =$ _____

6. $7 \times 10^{-3} =$ _____

Solve.

7. Blood is carried from your heart to the rest of your body through a complex network of vessels. These vessels measure more than 9.65×10^4 kilometers. What is the approximate length of these vessels in kilometers written in standard form? _____

8. The average adult eye ball is about 0.024 meters long. Write this length in scientific notation. _____

Square Roots

The square root sign is $\sqrt{}$. To find the square root of a number (x), one finds the factor that when multiplied by itself one time equals the number (x) inside the square root sign. For example, $\sqrt{100}$. $10 \times 10 = 100$ or 10^2. Thus, the square root of $\sqrt{100}$ is 10. This is called a perfect square because the factors are whole numbers.

Practice Determine the square root for each.

1. $\sqrt{16}$ _____

2. $\sqrt{36}$ _____

3. $\sqrt{81}$ _____

4. $\sqrt{225}$ _____

5. $\sqrt{121}$ _____

6. $\sqrt{49}$ _____

7. $\sqrt{196}$ _____

8. $\sqrt{256}$ _____

9. $\sqrt{289}$ _____

10. $\sqrt{64}$ _____

Order of Operations

Mathematicians have developed a standard order of operations for calculations that have more than one arithmetic operation. Following the order of operation allows for only one correct answer for each problem.

Step 1: Perform any calculations inside parentheses, fraction bars, exponents and square roots.

Step 2: Perform all multiplications and divisions, working from left to right.

Step 3: Perform all additions and subtractions, working from left to right

> Some instructors use the mnemonic device "Please excuse my Dear Aunt Sally" (PEMDAS) to help students remember the correct order.
> P: Parentheses and fraction bars
> E: Exponents and roots
> M: { Multiplication
> D: { Division
> A: { Addition
> S: { Subtraction

In the following example, we can see why the order of operation is helpful.

$$5 + 7 \times 8 = \underline{\quad}$$

Following the order of operations (PEMDAS),

Step 1: $7 \times 8 = 56$

Step 2: $56 + 5 = 61$

If the order of operations is not followed, the answer would incorrectly come out to $5 + 7 = 12$ and $12 \times 8 = 96$. Thus, the value of having a rule to follow to ensure following a set pattern for calculating each operation is important.

Practice Solve the following operations.

1. $(4 \times 5) \times 2 = \underline{\quad}$

2. $8 + 9 - (3 \times 2) = \underline{\quad}$

3. $(5 \times 3) - 8 \div 2 = \underline{\quad}$

4. $4 \times (12 - 8) + 3 = \underline{\quad}$

5. $(500 - 250) \div 25 + 1 = \underline{\quad}$

6. $(24 \div 3) \times 2 + 12 = \underline{\quad}$

7. $10 - 6 \times (14 \div 2) = \underline{\quad}$

8. $\dfrac{(124 \div 4)}{1} =$ _____

9. $\dfrac{(15 \times 3)}{(5 \times 1)} =$ _____

10. $352 - (34 - 2) + 2 \times 14 =$ _____

Algebraic Expressions

A variable is a letter or symbol that represents an unknown number. Letters such as p, t, x or y are used to represent variables. For example, we can use s to stand for the number of students when calculating the cost of educating a class of nurses for a year. A variable can be used in addition, subtraction, multiplication and/or division problems. Some variables have coefficients like the -8 in $-8s$, where the coefficient or number -8 is multiplied by the unknown number s. If a variable appears by itself as s, or xy, it is understood to have a coefficient of 1 because $s = 1s$ and $xy = 1xy$.

Expressions

An expression is a mathematical statement that may use numbers and/or variables. An algebraic expression is an expression that contains one or more variables.

The following are examples of expressions:

Examples

$$9 + z$$
$$xy$$
$$9(3 - r)$$
$$20 + (9 - x)$$

An expression is also used to build a mathematical statement from words as in a word problem.

An LPN spends \$240.00 on books and a dental assistant spends y on books. Write an expression for their combined amounts of dollars spent on books. The combined amount of an LPN's spending to a dental assistant's spending is \$240.00 + y.

Practice For each problem, identify the variable and the coefficient.

	Expression	Variable	Coefficient
1	$2a^3$		
2	$5bcd$		
3	$1.5x$		
4	$7z^2$		
5	$12ab^2c$		
6	$22xy$		
7	$2bc^3$		
8	$-xyz$		
9	$-7bc$		
10	abc		

To evaluate an expression at some number means we replace or substitute a variable in an expression with the number, and simplify the expression. Some common algebraic expressions are

some number n increased by 2.7 $\rightarrow n + 2.7$

9 less than some number $x \rightarrow x - 9$

The sum of two numbers a and $b \rightarrow a + b$

some number q multiplied by 5 $\rightarrow 5q$

the product of x and $-9 \rightarrow -9x$

4 times the sum of three numbers $x, y,$ and $z \rightarrow 4(x + y + z)$

The sum of two numbers y and z divided by $-8 \rightarrow \dfrac{y + z}{-8}$

Note: the variable is always written after the numeral.

Practice   Write the algebraic expression for each mathematical statement.

Word phrase	**Algebraic expression**
some number c decreased by 1.5	_____
some number z multiplied by 3	_____
the sum of two numbers a and b	_____
some number x divided by 5	_____
the sum of two numbers a and b divided by 6	_____
five times the sum of two numbers x and y	_____
the quotient of some number r and 3	_____
six less than some number x	_____
the sum of two numbers m and n multiplied by 2	_____
the sum of some number x and 24	_____

Practice   Write an algebraic expression in words for each number statement.

1. $a + b - z$ _____

2. $w(y + 2)$ _____

3. $\dfrac{x}{y} - 15$ _____

4. $125 \div (35 - 10)$ _____

5. $7ab - 15$ _____

Algebraic expressions are not *solved* as in computation, but instead they are *evaluated*. The value of the variable is often given and it is used to replace the variable in the expression.

For example, evaluate the expression $5 \cdot y + 12$ when y equals 12.

Step 1: Replace z with 12. $5 \cdot 12 + 12$

Step 2: Follow order of operation steps

$$5 \cdot 12 = 60 \text{ (multiply first)}$$

$$60 + 12 = 72 \text{ (then add)}$$

The algebraic expression equals 72.

Evaluate the expression using substitution.

$$(4 + x) \times 2 + 15 \div 3 - x \quad \text{when } x = 2.$$

We replace each occurrence of x with the number 2, and simplify applying the usual order of operation rules: parentheses first, then exponents, multiplication and division, and finally addition and subtraction.

$(4 + x) \times 2 + 15 \div 3 - x$	First, replace each x with 2 so the expression becomes
$(4 + 2) \times 2 + 15 \div 3 - 2 =$	Next handle the parenthesis
$6 \times 2 + 15 \div 3 - 2 =$	Then multiply and divide
$12 + 5 - 2 =$	Complete the addition and subtraction
$17 - 2 = 15$	

Practice Use substitution to evaluate these expressions. Let $a = 5$, $b = 4$, and $c = 1$.

1. $4a^2$

2. $5a^2b$

3. $2a + b^2c^0$

4. $7ca^2$

5. $3b - c^2$

Practice Evaluate each expression.

1. $35 - \dfrac{(3 \cdot 7)}{4} =$

2. $\dfrac{(7 + 33)}{4 \div 2} =$

3. $\dfrac{3}{4}(10 - 4) =$

4. $\dfrac{1}{2}(8) + \dfrac{1}{4}(24) =$

Evaluate each expression if $x = 5$, $y = 10$, and $z = 15$.

5. $\frac{1}{2}(8y) =$

6. $\frac{3}{4}(6 - x) =$

7. $6z - y =$

8. $(z - x)(x + 5) =$

9. $\frac{(y - z)}{5} =$

10. $x(y + z - 4) =$

Writing Expressions from Word Problems

The most important use of writing expressions is in real life situations. Careful reading of the problem will help you ensure that you use the correct mathematical operation.

Here are some key words to help guide you:

=	+	−	×	÷
is	add	subtract	multiply	divide
as	sum	difference	product	quotient
equals	plus	minus	times	split
equal to	total	remainder	"of"	per
	more than	less than		
	increased by	decreased by		

Reading word problems takes attention to detail. Sometimes, there can be confusion over some expressions.

For instance, "five more than x", which is written $x + 5$ and "five is more than x" which is written $5 > x$ look very similar. The difference here is the word "is". "$x + 5$" is an expression, not an equation or inequality like "$5 > x$".

Here is another example, "four less than z" which should be written $z - 4$, not $4 - z$ or $4 < z$. "$4 - z$" would be written four minus z. And the equation or inequality "$4 < z$" would be written four is less than z.

For example, how would you write an expression to represent that you got twelve points higher on this anatomy test than the last one?

First, choose and define your variable:

Let $x =$ the score you got on the last test.

So the expression to show twelve more is $x + 12$.

Here are some more examples:

a. There are twice the number of LPNs to the number of RNs on this shift. You could express this statement as 2*p*.

b. The insurance rate for eye care has increased by $250.00. (*x* + 250)

c. The shift has ten fewer patients to care for. (*r* − 10)

d. This nursing supervisor has three more than twice as many years of experience as the former supervisor. (2*s* + 3)

Practice   Write an expression to represent each word problem.

1. Robert had two fewer cavities than I had. _____

2. I doubled my income after I finished the certificate program. _____

3. The stipend increased her income by 500 dollars. _____

4. Dr. Phil Berg has five more than twice the number of patients than any other dentist. _____

5. He lost 12 pounds this month. _____

Solving Equations

To solve an equation, get the variable by itself on one side of the equal to sign. Use inverse operations to do this:

- addition is the inverse of subtraction and vice versa.

- multiplication is the inverse of division and vice versa.

Here are some examples.

Solve the equation: $x + 1.5 = -5.2$

$x + 1.5 - 1.5 = -5.2 - 1.5$ To get x by itself on the left side of the equation, subtract 1.5 from both sides of the equation.

$x = -6.7$ Simplify each side.

Solve the equation: $z - 7 = 5$

$z - 7 + 7 = 5 + 7$ To get z by itself on the left side of the equation, add the 7 to both sides of equation.

$z = 12$ Simplify each side.

Solve the equation $5a = 36$

$$\frac{5a}{5} = \frac{36}{5}$$ To get a by itself on the left side of the equation, divide both sides by 5.

$a = 7.2$ or $7\frac{1}{5}$ Simplify each side.

Solve the equation $\frac{y}{2} = 3.8$

$$\frac{y}{2} \cdot 2 = 3.8 \cdot 2$$ To get y by itself on the left side of the equation, multiply both sides by 2.

$y = 7.6$ or $7\frac{3}{5}$ Simplify each side.

Practice   Solve the equations.

1. $x + 7.5 = 65$

2. $z - 13 = 42$

3. $k + 3\frac{1}{2} = 45$

4. $r - 5 = 17.4$

5. $b - 4.25 = -16.5$

6. $-6a = -4.5$

7. $\frac{t}{-8} = 16.2$

8. $12c = 60$

9. $\frac{m}{4} = -4.1$

10. $-50w = -14$

Writing Equations from Word Problems

An algebraic equation is an equation that contains one or more variables. There will also be algebraic expressions on both sides of the equation. So an equation is a mathematical sentence with an equal sign that illustrates that two expressions represent the same number. To accomplish this, you must be able to translate word sentences or other data into equations.

If the patient's temperature decreased by 2 degrees, it will be 99.4 degrees. What is the patient's temperature now?

Use t for the variable representing the patient's temperature

temperature decreased by 2 degrees is 99.4 degrees
$$\downarrow \qquad \downarrow \qquad \downarrow \qquad \downarrow\ \downarrow$$
$$t \qquad - \qquad 2 \qquad =\ 99.4$$

Solve the equation: $t - 2 = 99.4$

$t - 2 + 2 = 99.4 + 2$ To get t by itself on the left side of the equation, add the 2 to both sides of the equation.

$t = 101.4$ Simplify.

If a certified nurse's aid works a 12-hour shift, he or she will earn $165. How much will the aid make in an hour?

Use x for the amount that the aid earns each hour.

12 hours times the amount earned per hour is $165.
12   times x = $165
$12x = 165$

Solve the equation: $12x = 165$

$$\frac{12x}{12} = \frac{165}{12}$$ Divide both sides by 12.

$$x = 13.75$$ Simplify.

Practice   Write an equation to represent each word problem. Then solve it.

1. Sharon wants to donate 123 nursing books to the college library. The nursing collection has 1,357 books stored on the library shelves. How many books will be in the collection after Sharon's donation?

   Equation: _____   Solution: _____

2. If a patient's pulse decreases by 8 beats, it will be 78 beats a minute. How many beats a minute was the pulse before the decrease.

   Equation: _____   Solution: _____

3. If you double the cost of a dietitian's apron and then add $2, you will get the cost of a tailored dietitian's jacket. A dietitian's apron costs $16.50. How much will each dietitian's tailored jacket cost?

   Equation: _____   Solution: _____

4. The cost of a polymer crown is $1,005. The insurance pays $\frac{1}{2}$ the cost plus $75. What part of the bill is left for the patient to pay?

   Equation: _____   Solution: _____

5. Dinh has 7 more patients to care for than Juan. If Dinh has 18 patients to care for, how many does Juan have?

   Equation: _____   Solution: _____

6. If you divide a number by 5 and add −8, the result is 3. What is the number?

   Equation: _____   Solution: _____

7. If you multiply a number by 4 and add 7, the result is the 31 residents who work in the large city hospital. What is the number?

   Equation: _____   Solution: _____

8. Together the surgical technicians spend $112.44 for lunch. There were 12 technicians. How much did each spend on lunch?

   Equation: _____   Solution: _____

9. The cost of an eye appointment is $125 and imported frames are $325. If the patient paid a total of $625.35, what is the cost of the lens and the coatings?

Equation: _____   Solution: _____

10. The sum of a number and 3 times the same number is 100. What is the number?

Equation: _____   Solution: _____

Literal Equations

A literal equation has one term that is defined by other terms and/or numbers. You might have seen these in mathematical formulas and not known what they are called. Literal equations are solved changing the formula around to solve for an unknown. You will be solving the equation for one of the variables. To accomplish this, move all the letters away from the one you are solving for by applying two rules of algebra.

Rule 1: Isolate the unknown on one side of the equation using the opposite or inverse operation(s). (The opposite of + is − and the opposite of × is ÷.)

Rule 2: Whatever math function is completed on one side of the equation must be done to the other side of the equation.

A commonly used formula in health care is IV flow rate

$$R = \frac{V}{t}$$

This means that the flow rate (R) may be solved in terms of drug volume (V) and time (t).

For example, you are asked to solve for volume (V). You must isolate V to solve the literal equation.

Apply rule 1: Use the inverse operation. To find V, multiply both sides by t to isolate the variable.

In our equation, $R = V/_t$, V is divided by t. To isolate V, we will use the inverse operation of division, which is multiplication.

So our equation changes to be

$$R = \frac{V}{t} \rightarrow R = \frac{V(t)}{t}$$

Apply rule 2: Perform the same function on both sides of the equation.

$$R(t) = \frac{V(t)}{t}$$

Now, apply cancellation of like units. Volume is now solved in terms of $V = R(t)$ or $R(t) = V$.

These types of formulas will be used in Unit 13 for completing a variety of IV drug administration flow rates.

Practice   Rewrite these common formulas as literal equations in terms of the unknown.

1. Rewrite the interest formula, $i = pt$, in terms of t.

2. Rewrite the distance formula, $d = rt$, in terms of t.

3. Rewrite the perimeter formula, $p = 4s$, in terms of s.

4. Rewrite the area formula, $a = lw$, in terms of w.

5. Rewrite $B = \dfrac{W}{H}$ in terms of W.

PRE-ALGEBRA BASICS SELF-TEST

1. $-6 + 5 = $ _____

2. $-12 - 12 = $ _____

3. $5 + 4 \times 8 - 16 \div 4 = $ _____

4. $12 - 40 \div 2 \div 5 + 2 = $ _____

5. $4^2 + 3^0 = $ _____

6. $12^3 \times 3^2 = $ _____

7. $\sqrt{121} = $ _____

8. $\sqrt{9} \times 20 = $ _____

9. $|-68| = $ _____

10. $10 - 8 \times 2 + 12 \div 3 = $ _____

11. The coefficient of $ab4f$ is _____

12. Write as an expression: the quotient of some number y and 5
_____

13. Solve: $\dfrac{t}{-4} = 24.4$ _____

14. Beth has $450 more than Fred. Together they have $3,219. How much money does Fred have? _____

15. Subtract 10 from Thanh's age and double the result, and you get Xuyen's age. Xuyen is 22. How old is Thanh? _____

Unit 8

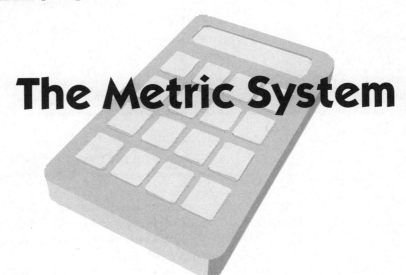

The Metric System

Metric measurements are used for many types of measurements in the health care professions. Some uses include the following:

- weight calculations
- dosage calculations
- food intake (in grams) measurements
- height and length measurements
- liquid and medication measurements

Metric units come in base units. These units measure different types of materials.

Base unit	Measurement type	Examples
Liter	volume	liquids, blood, urine
Gram	weight	an item's weight
		an amount of medicine
Meter	length	height, length, instruments

The metric system uses units based on multiples of ten. For this reason, metric numbers are written in whole numbers or decimal numbers, never fractions. Metric conversion problems can be solved by moving the decimal either to the left or to the right. This chart resembles the decimal place value chart on page 160. Review the similarities.

Unit:	kilo-	hecto-	deka	base	deci	centi-	milli-	x	x	micro
Value:	1,000	100	10	1 meter (m)	0.1	0.01	0.001			0.000001
Symbol:	k	h	da	grams (g) liter (l or L)	d	c	m			mc or μ
Mnemonic Device:	kiss	hairy	dogs	but	drink	chocolate	milk,	m	o	m

> Decimals and metric measurements are based on units of ten.

Using a mnemonic device helps keep the metric units in the correct sequence or order. Try something silly like "kiss hairy dogs but drink chocolate milk, mom." Knowing a device like this will help you remember the order of the units on an exam.

Note that the *mo* are placeholders. This helps one remember to count the spaces in the mnemonic device.

Using the Metric Symbols

The metric system uses the unit of measure, a prefix, and a base element to form the metric units. To form *millimeter*, take *m* from *milli* and *m* from meter and form *mm*, which represents the *millimeter*.

The metric system combines prefixes that give the unit and root words that indicate the type of measurement, as in volume, weight, or length. The prefixes are the key to deciphering what number of units you have.

Prefix	Meaning	Symbol
kilo-	thousand	k
hecto-	hundred	h
deka-	ten	da
base	one	m, g, L
deci-	tenth	d
centi-	hundredth	c
milli-	thousandth	m
micro-	millionth	mc or μ

Root	Use	Symbol
gram	weight	g
meter	length	m
liter	volume	L or l

Every metric prefix may be combined with every root. The application of these terms depends on the measurement being completed. Thus, liquids are measured in liters, and dry medication uses grams because this type of drug is measured by weight.

Supply the words or abbreviations:

1. kilogram	6. mm	11. km
2. mL	7. kilometer	12. meter
3. gram	8. mcg	13. microgram
4. mg	9. L	14. kL
5. centimeter	10. kg	15. cm

> k h d b d c m m o m

You can use the first letters of the metric units to recall their order by writing them on a piece of scratch paper or an answer sheet on examination days.

Changing Unit Measures

To change units within the metric system, review the number's place value and then consider where you are converting to. Count the number of spaces from the number you are starting with and the place you are converting to.

$$45.5 \text{ grams} = \underline{\hspace{1cm}} \text{ milligrams}$$

> k   h   d   b   d   c   m   m   o   m
> ← 3 spaces →   ← 3 spaces →   ← 3 spaces →

Note that the *mo* are placeholders. This helps one remember to count the spaces in the mnemonic device. Also, most conversions in health care are between the units of kilo (k), gram, meter, liter (b) and milli (m) and micro (m). There are three spaces to move between each of these to make the conversions.

From gram to milligram, there are three spaces. Note the direction from gram to milligram is to the right. Move the decimal three places to the right. Thus,

$$45.5 \text{ grams} = 45\,5\,0\,0 \text{ milligrams}$$

Note that most of the health care conversions are done between kilogram and gram, gram and milligram, milligram and microgram, meter and centimeter, and liter and milliliter. Once these are practiced, converting between units will feel natural. Practice making the conversion by moving the decimal from one unit to another. Use a pencil to draw the ∪ as you count the spaces. Start at the existing decimal and move to the right of each metric unit. Remember that "b" stands for the base units of meters, liters, or grams.

   In other fields, a cubic centimeter (cc) is viewed as a ▢, but in health care professions a cubic centimeter is the same as milliliter. The logic for this is that a syringe has a tube and measures volume in cc or ml. Thus, cubic centimeter equals milliliter.

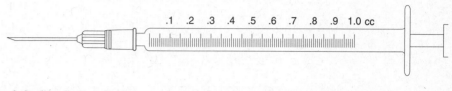

1. k h d b d c m m o m   4 grams = _____ kilogram

2. k h d b d c m m o m   360 grams = _____ milligrams

3. k h d b d c m m o m   9.25 kilograms = _____ grams

4. k h d b d c m m o m   220 cubic centimeters = _____ liters

5. k h d b d c m m o m   _____ gram = 1000 micrograms

6. k h d b d c m m o m   _____ milligram = 426 micrograms

7. k h d b d c m m o m   _____ kilogram = 358.6 grams

8. k h d b d c m m o m   _____ centimeters = 3.97 meters

9. k h d b d c m m o m   37.5 micrograms = _____ milligrams

10. k h d b d c m m o m   _____ centimeter = 6.75 millimeters

   Use these letters and the mnemonic device as a quick memory tool for test recall or assignments.

Example   Use as work space with the mnemonic device.

   50 milliliters = _____ liter   k h d b d c m m o m

   0.0 5 0
     ∪∪∪ = 0.05 liter

Practice   1. 1 cubic centimeter = _____ milliliter

   2. 0.5 liter = _____ milliliter

   3. _____ milligram = 26 micrograms

4. 0.75 gram = _____ milligrams

5. 19.5 kilograms = _____ grams

6. 15 milligrams = _____ gram

7. _____ grams = 0.3 kilogram

8. 8.5 liter = _____ milliliters

9. 0.07 milligram = _____ micrograms

10. 4 kilograms = _____ milligrams

11. 14 centimeters = _____ meter

12. 0.001 kilogram = _____ gram

13. _____ liter = 250 cubic centimeters

14. 3.8 milligrams = _____ gram

15. _____ milligrams = 0.6 gram

16. 56.75 milliliters = _____ liter

17. _____ milligram = 36 grams

18. _____ gram = 10 milligrams

19. 7500 milliliters = _____ liters

20. _____ millimeters = 50 centimeters

Additional Practice

Unit:	kilo-	hecto-	deka	base	deci	centi-	milli-	x	x	micro
Value:	1,000	100	10	1 meter (m)	0.1	0.01	0.001			0.000001
Symbol:	k	h	da	grams (g) liter (L)	d	c	m			mc or μ
Mnemonic Device:	kiss	hairy	dogs	but	drink	chocolate	milk,	m	o	m

21. 12.5 milligrams = _____ micrograms

22. 5.78 grams = _____ kilogram

23. 24 decimeters = _____ centimeters

24. 250 micrograms = _____ milligram

25. 12.76 kilograms = _____ grams

26. 45 meters = _____ millimeters

27. 23.5 centimeters = _____ millimeters

28. 750 micrograms = _____ milligram

29. 800 centimeters = _____ meters

30. 0.0975 milligram = _____ micrograms

31. 1000 milliliters = _____ liter

32. 3 kilograms = _____ grams

33. 12500 centimeters = _____ meters

34. 75.5 milligrams = _____ micrograms

35. 0.125 gram = _____ milligrams

36. 0.150 milligram = _____ microgram

37. 45250 milligram = _____ gram

38. 9500 grams = _____ kilograms

39. 1000 micrograms = _____ gram

40. 25 microgram = _____ milligram

41. 5524 grams = _____ kilograms

42. 45 milliliters = _____ liter

43. 1.25 meters = _____ centimeters

44. 550 micrograms = _____ milligram

45. 0.09 liter = _____ milliliters

46. 24.5 centimeters = _____ meter

47. 0.1 gram = _____ milligrams

48. 0.25 liter = _____ milliliters

49. 8500 micrograms = _____ milligrams

50. 0.625 gram = _____ micrograms

Practice with Word Problems

1. The medical assistant was asked to measure the infant. The infant measured 0.4453 meters or _____ centimeters.

2. The client in the cardiac unit was asked to exercise on the treadmill. The physical assistant recorded 0.5 kilometers for the first day of physical therapy. The next day the client walked 0.68 kilometers. How many more meters did the client walk on the second day? _____

3. The nutritional aide noted that a plastic container of cranberry juice contained 1.89 liters. How many milliliters are in the bottle? _____ If the nutritional aide was asked to pour 180 milliliters servings from this container, how many full servings could be poured? _____

4. The medical assistant asked the client's family to ensure adequate fluid intake. She recommended at least 2.2 liters of fluids. How many milliliters would that be? _____ How many full 240 milliliters (8 ounce glasses) portions should the client drink a day? _____

5. The certified nurses aide measures the patient's output of urine to be 3100 milliliters. The patient is on a liquid diet and IV. In total, the patient has received 2.5 liters of dextrose water and drank a total of 1850 cubic centimeters of juice, water, tea, and broth. What is the difference in patient's intake from output in cubic centimeters? _____

6. A drug label notes that the client's medicine has 250 milligrams in 5 milliliters of syrup. How many milliliters would deliver 125 milligrams of medicine? _____

7. A child claims to have grown 3.5 centimeters since his last check up. His previous height was 1.2 meters. The medical assistant measures the child and discovers that he has grown 3.56 centimeters. What is the child's new recorded height in centimeters for his medical record? _____ What is the child's new recorded height in meters? _____

8. A can of pear halves weighs 425 grams. How many kilograms does the can weigh?

9. The pharmacy technician reads a prescription. The physician has ordered 0.03 grams of cevimeline hydrochloride for a client. The pharmacy has on hand 30 milligrams capsules. Is the physician's order consistent with the supply on hand in the pharmacy?_____ How do you know this? _____
_____.

10. Look at the following drug label.

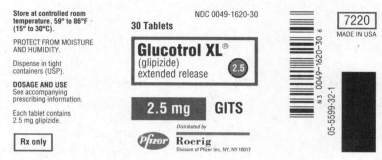

Used with permission from Pfizer, Inc.

How many micrograms are given in each tablet? _____

METRIC SYSTEM SELF-TEST

1. Look at the drug label. How many micrograms are in 5 milliliters of Neurontin? _____

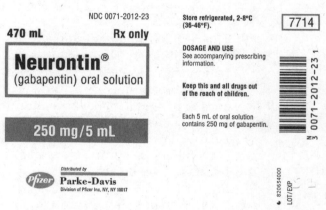

Used with permission from Pfizer, Inc.

2. _____ milligrams = 75 micrograms

3. _____ kilogram = 54.6 grams

4. 8.3 liters = _____ cubic centimeters

5. 0.014 gram = _____ micrograms

6. 1.2 milliliters = _____ liter

7. 10 micrograms = _____ gram

8. _____ liter = 250 cubic centimeter

9. _____ milligrams = 0.015 gram

10. _____ micrograms = 30 milligrams

11. 0.008 microgram = _____ milligram

12. The medical assistant was asked to measure the infant. The infant measured 0.345 meters or _____ centimeters.

13. A drug label notes that the client's medicine has 250 milligrams in 5 milliliters of syrup. How many milliliters would deliver 375 milligrams of medicine? _____

14. The pharmacy technician aide noted that a plastic container of medication contained 0.24 liter. How many milliliters are in the bottle? _____

15. 0.75 gram = _____ milligrams

Unit 9

Reading Drug Labels, Medicine Cups, Syringes, and Intravenous Fluid Administration Bags

Reading medication labels is part of the workplace skills for the allied health career. Most prescription drug labels contain certain information:

Name	Information presented
Generic name	Indicates that the drug is not protected by trademark; it is the nonproprietary name.
Trade name	Indicates the brand name; may have a ® or ™.
Manufacturer	Indicates the maker or manufacturer of the drug.
National Drug Code (NDC) number	Identifies the manufacturer, medication, and the container size.
Lot number (control number)	Placed on the label prior to shipping to identify the lot.
Drug form	Indicates cream, capsule, caplet, drop, tablet, suppository, syrup, etc.
Dosage strength	Provides the strength per dose as in tablet, milliliter, syrup, etc.
Usual adult dose	Indicates the usual adult dose for typical use.
Total amount in vial, packet, box	Indicates the total number of items in the container.
Prescription warning	Indicates that the medication is a prescription drug.
Expiration date	Provides the last date that the medication should be taken, applied, or used.

Example

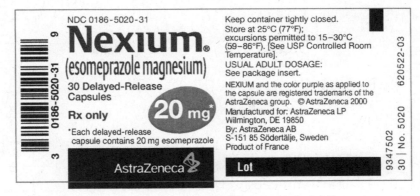

Used with permission from AstraZeneca Pharmaceuticals LP

Generic name	Esomeprazole magnesium
Trade name	Nexium
Manufacturer	AstraZeneca
National Drug Code (NDC) number	0186-5022-28
Lot number (control number)	Not shown*
Drug form	Capsules
Dosage strength	20 milligrams
Usual adult dose	See package insert
Total amount in vial, packet, box	100 Delayed-release capsules
Prescription warning	Rx only
Expiration date	Not shown

*The lot number and expiration date occur on actual prescriptions. These labels are educational and thus these labels do not show this information.

Practice

1. Complete the table for this drug label. If the information is not provided, write *not shown*.

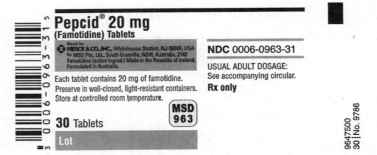

The labels for the products Prinivil, Fosamax, Singulair, Cozaar, Pepcid, Hyzaar, and Zocor are reproduced with the permission of Merck & Co., Inc., copyright owner.

Generic name   _____

Trade name   _____

Manufacturer   _____

National Drug Code (NDC) number   _____

Lot number (control number)   _____

Drug form   _____

Dosage strength   _____

Usual adult dose   _____

Total amount in vial, packet, box   _____

Prescription warning   _____

Expiration date   _____

2. Complete the table for this drug label. If the information is not provided, write *not shown*.

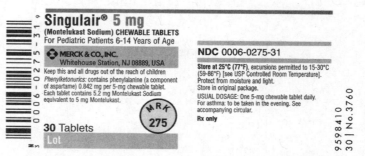

The labels for the products Prinivil, Fosamax, Singulair, Cozaar, Pepcid, Hyzaar, and Zocor are reproduced with the permission of Merck & Co., Inc., copyright owner.

Generic name   _____

Trade name   _____

Manufacturer   _____

National Drug Code (NDC) number   _____

Lot number (control number)   _____

Drug form   _____

Dosage strength   _____

Usual adult dose   _____

Total amount in vial, packet, box   _____

Prescription warning   _____

Expiration date   _____

3. Complete the table for this drug label. If the information is not provided, write *not shown*.

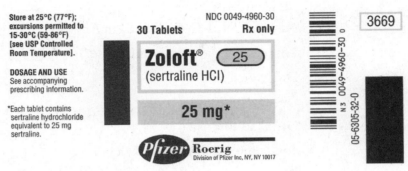

Store at 25°C (77°F); excursions permitted to 15-30°C (59-86°F) [see USP Controlled Room Temperature].

DOSAGE AND USE
See accompanying prescribing information.

*Each tablet contains sertraline hydrochloride equivalent to 25 mg sertraline.

NDC 0049-4960-30
30 Tablets   Rx only
Zoloft® (25)
(sertraline HCl)
25 mg*

Pfizer Roerig
Division of Pfizer Inc, NY, NY 10017

3669

N 3 0049-4960-30 0
05-6305-32-0

Used with permission from Pfizer, Inc.

Generic name _____

Trade name _____

Manufacturer _____

National Drug Code (NDC) number _____

Lot number (control number) _____

Drug form _____

Dosage strength _____

Usual adult dose _____

Total amount in vial, packet, box _____

Prescription warning _____

Expiration date _____

4. Complete the table for this drug label. If the information is not provided, write *not shown*.

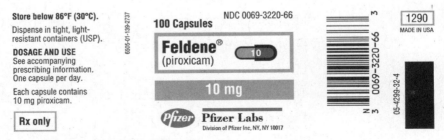

Store below 86°F (30°C).

Dispense in tight, light-resistant containers (USP).

DOSAGE AND USE
See accompanying prescribing information.
One capsule per day.

Each capsule contains 10 mg piroxicam.

Rx only

6505-01-139-2737

NDC 0069-3220-66
100 Capsules
Feldene® (10)
(piroxicam)
10 mg

Pfizer **Pfizer Labs**
Division of Pfizer Inc, NY, NY 10017

1290
MADE IN USA

N 3 0069-3220-66 3
05-4299-32-4

Used with permission from Pfizer, Inc.

Generic name   _____

Trade name   _____

Manufacturer   _____

National Drug Code (NDC) number   _____

Lot number (control number)   _____

Drug form   _____

Dosage strength   _____

Usual adult dose   _____

Total amount in vial, packet, box   _____

Prescription warning   _____

Expiration date   _____

5. Complete the table for this drug label.

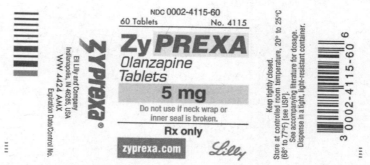

©Copyright Eli Lilly and Company. All rights reserved. Used with permission. ®HUMULIN, ®EVISTA, ®ZYPREXA are registered trademarks of Eli Lilly and Company.

Generic name   _____

Trade name   _____

Manufacturer   _____

National Drug Code (NDC) number   _____

Lot number (control number)   _____

Drug form   _____

Dosage strength   _____

Usual adult dose   _____

Total amount in vial, packet, box   _____

Prescription warning   _____

Expiration date   _____

Medicine cups are used to dispense liquid medications such as cough syrup and Maalox or milk of magnesia. The solution is poured into the medicine cup. The reading is made from a level counter top to ensure accuracy.

For example, the nurse read the order: Give 20 milliliters of cough syrup every 4 to 6 hours as needed. She will pour 20 milliliters into the medicine cup for her client.

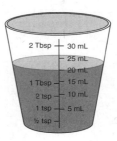

Practice   Read the following medicine cups and note the volume of medication.

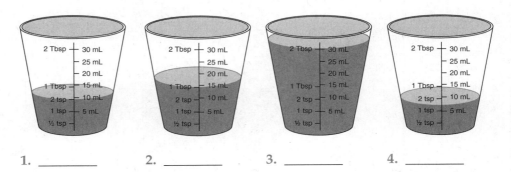

1. _____   2. _____   3. _____   4. _____

Syringes are labels in tenths and hundredths. The barrel of the syringe has markings in milliliters (mL), or units. Sometimes cubic centimeter (cc) and minim (*m*) are used. The units indicate volume. Carefully read the syringe from the edge of the plunger closest to the needle.

Example

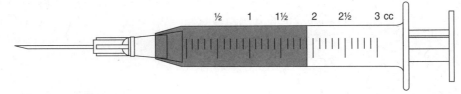

1.9 cubic centimeters

Practice   Read the following syringes and indicate the total volume of the solution in each syringe.

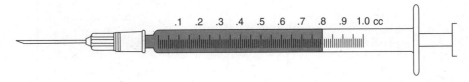

1. _____

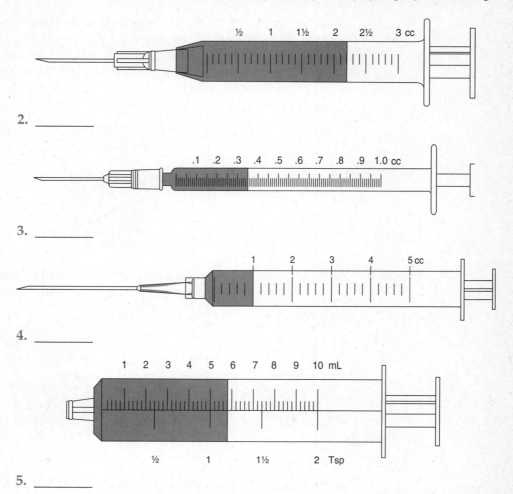

2. _____

3. _____

4. _____

5. _____

Determining the amount of liquid remaining in an IV bag is straightforward. Most IV bags today are made from durable plastic. Intravenous bags are supplied in a variety of sizes: 250 mL, 500 mL, and 1,000 mL. Smaller bags are available for mixing specific medications and these come in 100 mL. The capacity is noted on the bag. The bag is read by subtracting the volume of the infused fluid from the capacity noted on the bag.

For example, look at this 500 milliliters bag. Observe that 200 milliliters has been infused.

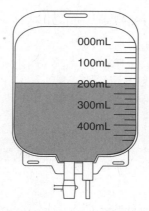

So, 500 milliliters − 200 milliliters = 300 milliliters remained to be infused.

Practice Note the volume of IV fluid infused and remaining to be infused.

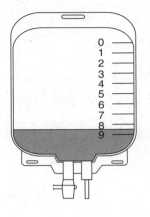

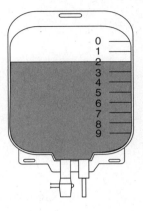

1. Volume infused _____
   Volume remaining _____

2. Volume infused _____
   Volume remaining _____

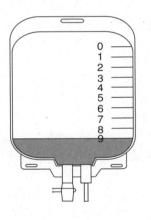

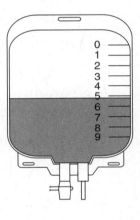

3. Volume infused _____
   Volume remaining _____

4. Volume infused _____
   Volume remaining _____

READING DRUG LABELS, MEDICINE CUPS, SYRINGES, AND IV FLUID ADMINISTRATION BAGS SELF-TEST

1. Explain the difference between the generic name and the trade name of a prescription medication.

   _____

   _____

   _____

   _____

2. Look at the label and provide the following information:

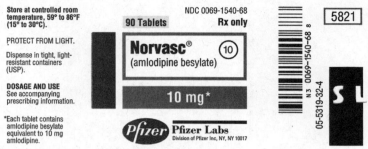

Used with permission from Pfizer, Inc.

Generic name _____

Trade name _____

Manufacturer _____

National Drug Code (NDC) number _____

Lot number (control number) _____

Drug form _____

Dosage strength _____

Usual adult dose _____

Total amount in vial, packet, box _____

Prescription warning _____

Expiration date _____

3. The medical assistants were asked to dispense 7.5 milliliters of a liquid medication. Shade the medicine cup to indicate this dosage.

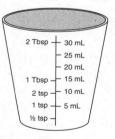

4. The physician has ordered an IM injection of 1.2 milliliters. Shade the syringe to indicate this volume of medication.

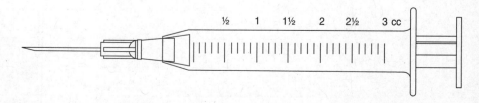

5. Volume infused _____
   Volume remaining _____

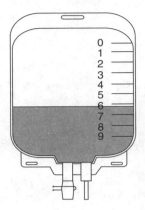

Unit 10

Apothecary Measurement and Conversion

This unit brings together the fundamental skills of the previous chapters and applies these basics to health care applications. Although new information is taught, the processes for arriving at the correct answers depend on your ability to compute using fractions, decimals, ratio, and proportion and, to a lesser degree, percents. This unit will cover the apothecary measurements and two methods of performing apothecary. These fundamentals will help prepare you for math applications in the health care professions.

Apothecary Measurement and Conversions

The apothecary system is a means for calculating drug amounts for medical fields. It relies on several number systems to denote measurements: lower case Roman numerals, Arabic numerals, and fractions. Some basic rules are applied in apothecary that do not exist in other measurement systems:

Rule 1: Fractions of $\frac{1}{2}$ may be written as *ss*.

Rule 2: Lower case Roman numerals are used for apothecary amounts of ten or less and for the numbers 20 and 30.

Rule 3: The symbol is placed before the quantity: Thus, grains $7\frac{1}{2}$ is written as *grains viiss* or *gr. viiss*.

In metric and household measurement, the symbol follows the quantity:

$$25 \text{ milligrams, } 3 \text{ cups, } 16\frac{1}{3} \text{ pounds.}$$

Check with your program instructor to learn if you will be using fractions or decimals in household weights.

Four common symbols that exist in apothecary need to be memorized:		
Term	**Symbol**	**Approximate Conversion**
fluid ounce	℥	fluid ounce 1 = drams 8
fluid dram	ℨ	dram 1 = 4 or 5 milliliters
minim	ℳ	
grain	gr.	grain i = 60 milligrams

Once you are familiar with these terms, symbols, and their equivalents, you will be ready to use these apothecary units in your conversions. This is a new concept for health care students to learn. We think of science and measurement as exact, but apothecary is a measurement system of approximate equivalents. Approximate equivalents come into play when you are converting among the measurement systems. Metric-to-metric or household-to-household measurement conversions usually can be done in exact measurements. In general, Metric- or household-to-apothecary measurement conversions are done through approximate measures. The equivalents are called approximate because they are rounded to the nearest whole number. In exact measures, 1 gram is equivalent to grains 15.432; however, the simple conversion in approximate equivalents used in health care is 1 gram = grains 15. To accomplish these conversions, you must memorize some of the approximate equivalents.

Approximate Equivalents

fluid dram 1 = 1 teaspoon
grain i = 60 milligrams
1 teaspoon = 5 milliliters
fluid ounce 1 = fluid drams 8
fluid ounce 1 = 2 tablespoons
fluid ounce 1 = 30 milliliters
1 quart = fluid ounces 32

1 inch = 2.54 centimeters
1 kilogram = 2.2 pounds
1 teaspoon = 60 drops

1 quart = 1 liter
1 cup = 240–250 milliliters

Notice that the conversions in the table are set up so that the unit (1) elements are all on the left and that these will be placed on top of the known part of the ratio and proportion equation. This simplifies the learning process, expedites learning, and helps recall of these conversions.

Practice These conversions are accomplished by setting up the known and unknown quantities in proportion format or with dimensional analysis.
Use the example below as your guide:

Example   How many milliliters are in $2\frac{1}{2}$ ounces?

To solve with proportion format:

    a. Set up the known conversion on one side of the equal sign and the unknown on the other side of the equal sign.

known   *unknown*

$$\frac{1 \text{ ounce}}{30 \text{ milliliters}} = \frac{2\frac{1}{2} \text{ ounces}}{? \text{ milliliters}}$$

    b. Cross multiply. $30 \times 2\frac{1}{2} = 75$

    c. Shortcut—any number divided by one is itself. Thus, the answer is 75 milliliters.

Example   Convert 48 milligrams to grains.

    a. Set up the known conversion on one side of the equal sign and the unknown on the other side of the equal sign.

known   *unknown*

$$\frac{\text{grain i gr}}{60 \text{ milligrams}} = \frac{? \text{ ounces}}{48 \text{ milligrams}}$$

    b. Cross multiply. $1 \times 48 = 48 \rightarrow \dfrac{48}{60}$

    c. Divide and/or reduce. $\dfrac{48}{60} \rightarrow$ reduces to grain $\dfrac{4}{5}$ gr

    The answer is grain $\dfrac{4}{5}$ gr

> **Hint:** Grains will be in whole numbers and/or fractions. Milliliters will be in whole numbers and decimals.

To solve with dimensional analysis:

How many milliliters are in $2\frac{1}{2}$ ounces?

    a. Place the unit of measure of the unknown on one side of the equation.

? milliliters =

    b. Use the conversion factor closest to the problem. Place the factor of the unit of measure for the answer on top and the units that you are converting to on the bottom as the denominator.

$$? \text{ milliliters} = \frac{30 \text{ milliliters}}{1 \text{ ounce}}$$

Hint: The first factor on the right side of the equation will have the same unit of measure as the unknown that is being solved for.

c. Multiply the first factor by the given information from the problem.

$$? \text{ milliliters} = \frac{30 \text{ milliliters}}{1 \text{ ounce}} \times \frac{2\frac{1}{2} \text{ ounces}}{1}$$

d. Cancel the like units and then solve by multiplication/division. Multiply straight across.

Hint: Units can only be cancelled if the same unit appears in both the numerator and the denominator. In other words, mL cancel mL, ounces cancel ounces. etc.

$$? \text{ milliliters} = \frac{30 \text{ milliliters}}{1 \text{ ounce}} \times \frac{2\frac{1}{2} \text{ ounces}}{1} \rightarrow 30 \text{ milliliters} \times 2\frac{1}{2}$$

$$= 75 \text{ milliliters}$$

The answer is 75 milliliters.

Example   Convert 48 milligrams to grains.

a. Place the unit of measure of the unknown on one side of the equation.

$$? \text{ grains} =$$

b. Use the conversion factor closest to the problem. Place the factor of the unit of measure for the answer on top and the units that you are converting to on the bottom as the denominator.

$$? \text{ grain} = \frac{\text{grain i gr}}{60 \text{ milligrams}}$$

Hint: The first factor on the right side of the equation will have the same unit of measure as the unknown that is being solved for.

c. Multiply the first factor by the given information from the problem. Multiply straight across.

$$? \text{ grain} = \frac{\text{grain i}}{60 \text{ milligrams}} \times \frac{48 \text{ milligram}}{1}$$

   d. Cancel the like units and then solve by multiplication/division.

$$? \text{ grain} = \frac{\text{grain i}}{60 \text{ milligrams}} \times \frac{48 \text{ milligrams}}{1} \rightarrow \frac{1 \times 48}{60 \times 1} =$$

   e. Reduce if necessary

$$\frac{48}{60} \rightarrow \text{reduces to grain } \frac{4}{5}$$

> **Hint:** Grains will be in whole numbers and/or fractions. Milliliters will be in whole numbers and decimals.

The answer is grain $\frac{4}{5}$

Practice   Conversions between metric and grains are dry equivalents. Use ratio and proportion or dimensional analysis. Show all of your work to the right of the problem.

   1. 30 milligrams = grain _____

   2. grain $\frac{1}{4}$ = _____ milligrams

   3. 75 milligrams = grains _____

   4. _____ milligram = grain $\frac{1}{150}$

   5. grain $\frac{1}{6}$ = _____ milligrams

   6. grain $\frac{1}{100}$ = _____ milligram

   7. 15 grams = grains _____

   8. 0.8 milligrams = grain _____

   9. grain _____ = 0.30 milligram

   10. 0.6 gram = grains _____

   11. grains iiiss = _____ milligrams

   12. 0.05 gram = grains _____

When completing multiple conversions, it is best to work within the same unit of measure before changing to another unit of measure. Do all of the metric conversions, then move to the grain conversions, or make the grain-to-metric conversion into milligrams, then convert from milligrams to grams or micrograms. By doing so, you will have only one math setup per problem. Use the standard conversion equivalents to make the conversions.

> microgram = mcg or μg (Note: mcg is the preferred form as μg may be misread.)

Practice

1. grains xv = _____ milligrams = _____ gram

2. 500 mg = grains _____ = _____ gram

3. 0.015 gram = grain _____ = _____ milligrams

4. 0.0001 gram = _____ milligram = grain _____

5. _____ milligram = _____ microgram = grain $\frac{1}{4}$

6. 0.3 milligram = grain _____ = _____ gram

7. grains iss = _____ milligrams = _____ gram

8. 400 micrograms = grain _____ = _____ milligram

9. grains viiiss = _____ milligrams = _____ grams

10. grain $\frac{1}{8}$ = _____ milligram

Liquid equivalents are converted in the same manner. A wider range of conversions are needed for these. Rely on the conversion charts, but work toward memorizing these equivalents so that you can efficiently apply them.

Practice Make these liquid conversions:

1. fluid ounce 1 = _____ teaspoons

2. 15 milliliters = fluid ounce _____

3. 1 tablespoon = _____ milliliters

4. 10 teaspoon = _____ milliliters

5. 6 teaspoons = fluid ounce _____

6. fluid ounce $\frac{1}{2}$ = _____ teaspoons

7. 45 milliliters = fluid ounces _____

8. 15 cubic centimeters = fluid ounce _____

9. 20 milliliters = _____ teaspoons

10. 3 tablespoons = _____ milliliters

11. $2\frac{1}{2}$ quarts = _____ milliliters

12. 45 milliliters = fluid ounces _____

13. 1 teaspoon = _____ cubic centimeters

14. $1\frac{1}{4}$ cup = _____ milliliters

15. 2 liters = fluid ounces _____

16. 2 tablespoons = fluid ounces _____

17. 15 teaspoons = _____ milliliters

18. 4 milliliters = _____ drops

19. 60 milliliters = _____ tablespoons

20. 2.5 milliliters = _____ teaspoon

Mixed Application   Make the following conversions:

1. grain $\frac{1}{2}$ = _____ milligrams

2. 2 teaspoons = _____ cubic centimeters

3. $12\frac{1}{2}$ teaspoons = _____ cubic centimeters

4. grain $\frac{1}{400}$ = _____ milligram

5. $2\frac{1}{4}$ quarts = _____ milliliters

6. 12 teaspoons = fluid ounces _____

7. fluid ounces 14 = _____ milliliters

8. 4.4 liters = _____ quarts

9. 35 cubic centimeters = _____ teaspoons

10. 30 milliliters = fluid ounce _____

11. grains viii = _____ milligrams

12. 4 kilograms = _____ pounds

13. 0.3 milligrams = grain _____

14. $39\frac{3}{5}$ pounds = _____ kilograms

15. $2\frac{1}{2}$ cups = fluid ounces _____

16. 250 milliliters = _____ pint

17. fluid ounces 4 = _____ cup

18. 15 milliliters = fluid ounce _____

19. grains v = _____ milligrams

20. 120 milligrams = grains _____

21. grain $\frac{1}{150}$ = _____ milligram

22. fluid ounce $\frac{1}{8}$ = fluid dram _____

23. $\frac{1}{4}$ cup = fluid ounces _____

24. fluid ounces 6 = _____ milliliters

25. grains vii = _____ milligrams

26. 16 tablespoons = fluid ounces _____

27. fluid ounces 6 = _____ tablespoons

28. 0.3 liter = fluid ounces _____

29. 14 inches = _____ centimeters

30. 90 milligrams = grains _____

31. fluid drams 40 = fluid ounces _____

32. 16 tablespoons = _____ milliliters

33. fluid ounces 3 = _____ tablespoons

34. grain $\frac{1}{100}$ = _____ micrograms

35. fluid ounces 64 = _____ pints

36. 0.4 milligram = grain _____

37. 5 teaspoon = _____ cubic centimeters

38. 75 milliliters = _____ tablespoons

39. $4\frac{1}{2}$ cups = fluid ounces _____

40. 90 milliliters = fluid ounces _____

Apothecary Conversions

Practice   Make these conversions:

1. 600 milligrams = grains _____

2. 180 milliliters = _____ tablespoons

3. 24 teaspoons = fluid ounce _____

4. fluid ounce $\frac{1}{2}$ _____ teaspoons

5. 5 tablespoons = _____ milliliters

6. fluid ounces 48 = _____ cups

7. 20 cubic centimeters = _____ teaspoons

8. third ounces 20 = _____ cups

9. grains xv = _____ milligrams

10. 750 milliliters = _____ pints

11. 240 cubic centimeters = fluid ounces _____

12. 0.3 milligram = _____ gram

13. $4\frac{1}{2}$ quarts = _____ milliliters

14. $6\frac{1}{2}$ teaspoons = _____ milliliters

15. 0.1 milligram = grain _____

16. 1500 milliliters = _____ cups

17. 4.5 liters = _____ quarts.

18. fluid ounces 96 = _____ liters

19. $1\frac{1}{4}$ cups _____ milliliters

20. 5 tablespoons = _____ teaspoons

21. fluid ounce 4 = _____ milliliters

22. 500 milligrams = grains _____

23. 120 milliliters = _____ teaspoons

24. $2\frac{1}{4}$ cups = _____ milliliters

25. $3\frac{1}{2}$ cups = _____ milliliters

Rounding in Dosage Calculations

The metric system is used to measure liquids, weights, and medicine. Rounding will make dealing with the applications more practical. To assist in this process, follow these three guidelines:

1. Any decimal number that stands alone without a whole number must have a 0 placed in the whole number place. This is the standard way of

noting a decimal number that does not have a whole number with it. It also helps ensure reading and interpreting the number correctly. Examples

$$0.5 \text{ gram} \quad 0.25 \text{ milligram} \quad 0.125 \text{ microgram}$$

2. Round decimals to the correct place value. This is somewhat dependent on your profession; however, some general guidelines exist. For example, kilogram and degrees in Celsius and Fahrenheit are placed in tenths.

3. Multi-step problems require that you convert between number systems, especially between fractions and decimals. If the drug measurement is in metrics (milligram, gram, microgram), the solution to the problem must be in decimals. There are no fractions in the metric system. There-fore, $\frac{1}{4}$ milligram is stated as 0.25 milligram.

> Correct formats mean correct answers!

Practice   Solve the problems below by using the three guidelines to ensure the correct format of these medications:

1. 25.89 kilograms

2. 2.7759 milliliters of liquid medicine

3. 12.54 milligrams of a tablet

4. $5\frac{1}{4}$ kilograms

5. $50\frac{1}{2}$ milligrams of pain medication

Additional Practice with Apothecary Conversions   Make the conversion and ensure accurate format of your answers.

1. 650 cubic centimeters = _____ pints

2. 20 minim = _____ milliliter

3. _____ teaspoon = 30 drops

4. grains v = _____ milligrams

5. $8\frac{1}{2}$ ounces = _____ cubic centimeters

6. 750 milliliters = _____ quarts

7. grains 15 = _____ gram

8. _____ milligrams = grain $\frac{1}{20}$

9. grains x = _____ milligrams

10. $7\frac{1}{2}$ teaspoons = _____ milliliters

11. grain $\frac{1}{6}$ = _____ milligrams

12. 98 pounds 8 ounces = _____ kilograms

13. 2 teaspoons = _____ drops

14. 400 milligrams = grains _____

15. $1\frac{1}{4}$ teaspoons = _____ drops

APOTHECARY SYSTEM SELF-TEST

1. Write seven and a half grains in medical notation. _____

2. 380 mg = grains _____

3. 0.3 mg = grain _____

4. grain iiss = _____ milligrams

5. fluid ounces 4 = _____ cubic centimeters

6. 48 kilograms = _____ pounds

7. 95 milliliters = _____ tablespoons

8. grain $\frac{1}{100}$ = _____ milligram

9. 75 milliliters = _____ fluid ounces

10. $1\frac{1}{2}$ milliliters = _____ drops

11. $7\frac{1}{2}$ fluid ounces = _____ milliliters

12. The client weighs $68\frac{1}{2}$ pounds. How many kilograms does this client weigh? _____

13. The physician's assistant prescribes 12 milliliters of cough syrup. How many teaspoons of cough syrup is that? _____

14. The residents in a weight reduction program are asked to drink eight 8-ounce glasses of water daily. How many milliliters of water is this per day? _____

15. Three ounces equals _____ milliliters.

Unit 11

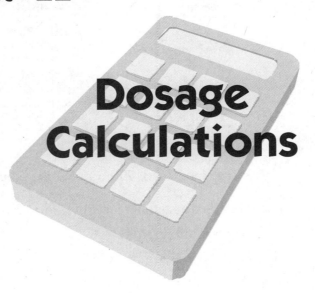

Dosage Calculations

This unit pulls together all the math skills reviewed and practiced previously in this text. Your task will be to determine the individual dose a client will receive.

In order to calculate an individual dose, one must know three important pieces of information: the desired dose, the dosage strength, and the medications' unit of measure. These are given in each dosage calculation.

Term	Symbol	Meaning	Example
dosage ordered or desired dose	D	the amount of medication that the physician has ordered for the client	Give 500 milligrams Give grains/v Give 1.2 milliliters
dosage strength or supply on hand	H	the amount of drug in a specific unit of measure	250 milligrams grains/v
unit of measure or quantity of unit	Q	the unit of measure for the specific dosage strength or supply on hand	_____ per 2 mL _____ per capsule _____ per tablet

We can see how these are used in the medication order:

The physician ordered Zithromax 500 milligrams once a day for his client.

The nurse looks at her medication label:

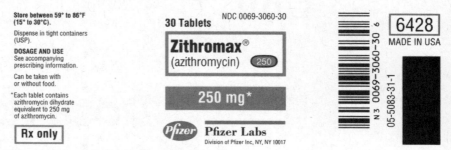

Used with permission from Pfizer, Inc.

The drug label reads Zithromax 250 milligrams per tablet.

The three essential pieces of information are

D = 500 milligrams

H = 250 milligrams

Q = 1 tablet

When using the dosage formula provided in this chapter, you must ensure that the medication information is in the correct place. This is true with any math formula. This formula can be used for most medication orders and is useful to memorize:

$$\frac{\text{desired or dosage ordered}}{\text{supply on hand}} \times \text{quantity} = \text{unknown dosage}$$

The formula is abbreviated as

$$\frac{D}{H} \times Q = x$$

Rule 1: The dosage ordered/desired and the have/supply must be in the same unit of measure.

Rule 2: The quantity and the unknown dosage will be in the same unit of measure.

Use the formula

$$\frac{\text{dosage(D)}}{\text{supply on hand(H)}} \times \text{quantity(Q)} = \text{medication given}$$

The dosage is the amount of the medication that the doctor orders. The supply on hand is the available form of the drug. In other words, milligrams, grams, caplets, tablets, and so on. This is what the pharmacy or the medication cabinet has on hand. The quantity is the amount of medication per tablet, milliliter, milligram, and so on.

It is important that the dosage and the supply on hand are in the same unit of measure. Thus, if the doctor's order is in milligrams, and you only have the medication in grams, you will convert the order to grams to match the supply that you have on hand.

You can apply this formula in two steps:

Example The doctor orders 250 milligrams. The supply in the medicine cabinet is in 125 milligrams tablets.

To solve with dosage calculation formula:

$$\frac{D}{H} \times Q = x \quad \begin{array}{l} \text{Order} = 250 \text{ milligrams} \\ \text{Have} = 125 \text{ milligrams} \end{array} \quad \text{quantity} = \begin{cases} \text{solid form of} \\ \text{medication, and} \\ \text{Q is 1, so Q can be} \\ \text{eliminated as a math} \\ \text{step in this problem.} \end{cases}$$

a. Put the information into the format

$$\frac{D}{H} \times Q = x \quad \frac{250 \text{ milligrams}}{125 \text{ milligrams}} \times 1 \text{ tablet} = X$$

b. Calculate. Remember that the horizontal line indicates division, so divide 250 by 125.

The result will be 2 tablets.

Example The doctor orders 60 milligrams of liquid cough syrup. The liquid cough syrup has a label that reads 100 milligrams in 5 milliliters.

a. Put the information into the format

$$\frac{D}{H} \times Q = x \rightarrow \frac{60 \text{ milliliters}}{100 \text{ milliliters}} \times 5 \text{ milliliters} = \underline{\quad} \text{ milliliters}$$

b. Multiply and divide.

$$\frac{60 \times 5}{100} = \frac{300}{100} =$$

c. Reduce to solve.

$$\frac{300}{100} = 3 \text{ milliliters}$$

The answer is 3 milliliters.

Example The doctor orders Zithromax 500 milligrams. The supply in the medicine cabinet is Zithromax 250 milligrams per tablet.

> Notice that the desired dose and the strength of the dosage supplied are in the same unit of measure. Thus, no conversion is needed.

a. Put the information into the format

$$\frac{D}{H} \times Q = x \rightarrow \frac{500 \text{ milligrams}}{250 \text{ milligrams}} \times 1 \text{ tablet} = \underline{\quad} \text{ tablets}$$

b. Multiply and divide.

$$\frac{500 \text{ milligrams}}{250 \text{ milligrams}} = 2 \text{ tablets}$$

The doctor orders Zithromax 500 milligrams. The supply in the medicine cabinet is Zithromax 250 milligrams per tablet.

> Notice that the desired dose and the strength of the dosage supplied are in the same unit of measure. Thus, no conversion is needed.

To solve with dimensional analysis

a. Place the unit of measure of the unknown on one side of the equation.

$$? \text{ tablets} =$$

b. The first factor is the unit of measure over the dosage strength.

$$? \text{ tablets} = \frac{1 \text{ tablet}}{250 \text{ milligrams}}$$

c. Multiply the first factor by the second, which is the dosage ordered over the number 1.

$$? \text{ tablets} = \frac{1 \text{ tablet}}{250 \text{ milligrams}} \times \frac{500 \text{ milligrams}}{1}$$

d. Cancel like units and multiply and divide.

$$? \text{ tablets} = \frac{1 \text{ tablet} \times 500}{250 \times 1} \quad \frac{500}{250} = 2 \text{ tablets}$$

The final answer is 2 tablets.

Example The doctor orders 60 milligrams of liquid cough syrup. The liquid cough syrup has a label that reads 100 milligrams in 5 milliliters.

a. Place the unit of measure of the unknown on one side of the equation

$$? \text{ milliliters} =$$

The first factor is the unit of measure over the dosage strength

$$? \text{ milliliters} = \frac{5 \text{ milliliters}}{100 \text{ milligrams}}$$

b. Multiply the first factor by the second, which is the dosage ordered over the number 1.

$$? \text{ milliliters} = \frac{5 \text{ milliliters}}{100 \text{ milligrams}} \times \frac{60 \text{ milligrams}}{1}$$

c. Cancel like units and multiply and divide.

$$? \text{ milliliters} = \frac{5}{100} \times \frac{60}{1} = \frac{300}{100} = 3 \text{ milliliters}$$

The final answer is 3 milliliters.

Practice   Choose a method of calculating dosage and complete the following dosage calculations:

1. Order: 30 milligrams
   Have: 10 milligrams per tablet
   Give: _____

2. Order: 1 milligram
   Have: 5 milligrams per milliliter
   Give: _____

3. Order: 1500 milligrams
   Have: 500 milligrams per tablet
   Give: _____

4. Order: 15 milligrams
   Have: 7.5 milligrams per tablet
   Give: _____

5. Order: 10 milligrams
   Have: 20 milligrams per milliliter
   Give: _____

6. Order: 0.25 gram
   Have: 50 milligrams in 2 milliliters
   Give: _____

7. Order: 1.5 milligrams
   Have: 3.0 milligrams per milliliter
   Give: _____

8. Order: 0.1 gram
   Have: 25 milligrams in 2 milliliters
   Give: _____

9. Order: 0.15 gram
    Have: 25 milligrams per tablet
    Give: _____

10. Order: 10 milligrams
    Have: 2.5 milligrams per capsule
    Give: _____

Now that the formula is familiar to you, the next step is to apply the metric and apothecary conversions you learned in this unit.

Convert the unit of measure of the "order" and "have" to the same unit of measure. One guideline is that it is often easier to convert the order to the have measure unit. This also helps in being able to compute the answer. Once the units are identifiable, it is easy to make the conversion. To review conversions among systems, reread Unit 13.

Practice

1. Order: 1 gram
    Have: 50 milligrams in 2 milliliters
    Give: _____

2. Order: 0.5 gram
    Have: 200 milligrams per tablet
    Give: _____

3. Order: 0.15 gram
    Have: 300 milligrams per caplet
    Give: _____

4. Order: grains x
    Have: 180 milligrams per milliliter
    Give: _____

5. Order: 0.06 gram
    Have: 15 milligrams per tablet
    Give: _____

6. Order: 1.5 gram
    Have: 125 milligrams per 2 milliliters
    Give: _____

7. Order: 1.5 grams
    Have: 1000 milligrams per tablet
    Give: _____

8. Order: grains iss
    Have: 30 milligrams per tablet
    Give: _____

9. Order: 1.5 gram
    Have: 750 milligrams per tablet
    Give: _____

10. Order: grain $\frac{1}{8}$
    Have: 7.5 milligrams per tablet
    Give: _____

More Dosage Calculation Practice

1. Order: 25 milligrams/orally
  Have: 10 milligrams scored tablets
  Give: _____

2. Order: 125 milligrams
  Have: 100 milligrams in 4 milliliters
  Give: _____

3. Order: grains iss
  Have: 50 milligrams per caplet
  Give: _____

4. Order: 75 milligrams
  Have: 25 milligrams in 2 milliliters
  Give: _____

5. Order: 25 milligrams/orally
  Have: 10 milligrams caplet
  Give: _____

6. Order: 300 milligrams
  Have: grains v in each tablet
  Give: _____

7. Order: 12.5 milliliters orally after meals
  Have: 25 milliliters
  Give: _____

8. Order: 0.25 milliliter by mouth
  Have: 0.125 milliliter
  Give: _____

9. Order: 120 milligrams by mouth
  Have: grain ss per tablet
  Give: _____

10. Order: 1500 milligrams
  Have: 500 milligrams per caplet
  Give: _____

Practice Using Drug Labels

Use the medication labels to complete these calculations. The drug label will supply the dosage strength and the unit.

1. The physician orders Glucotrol XL 10 milligrams once a day.

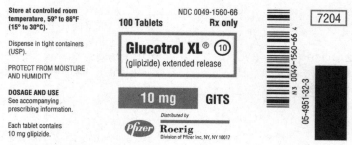

Used with permission from Pfizer, Inc.

Give: _____

2. The client has a medication order for Cozaar 50 milligrams once a day without food.

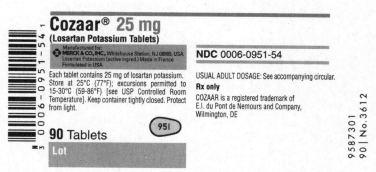

The labels for the products Prinivil, Fosamax, Singulair, Cozaar, Pepcid, Hyzaar, and Zocor are reproduced with the permission of Merck & Co., Inc., copyright owner.

Give: _____

3. The order is for Feldene 20 milligrams per day.

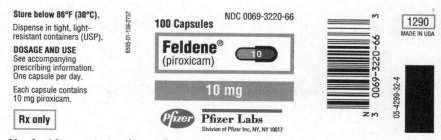

Used with permission from Pfizer, Inc.

Give: _____

$$4 \cdot (x-2) = 6 \cdot 3$$
$$6(x-2) = 4 \times 3$$

$$6(x-2) = 3 \times 4$$

4. The physician writes an order for Zoloft 25 milligrams per day.

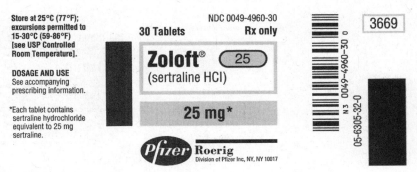

Used with permission from Pfizer, Inc.

Give: _____

5. Dr. Ballard writes an order for Procardia XL 60 milligrams once daily.

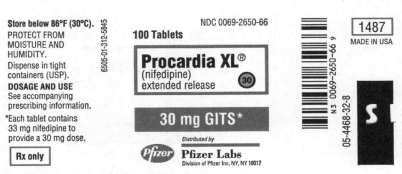

Used with permission from Pfizer, Inc.

Give: _____

6. The nurse receives a new order for Cardura XL 16 milligrams to control blood pressure.

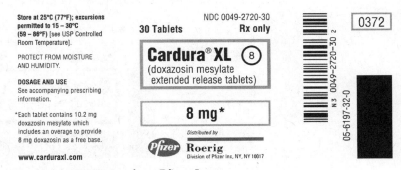

Used with permission from Pfizer, Inc.

Give: _____

7. The physician has written an order for Dilantin 100 milligrams chewable tablets.

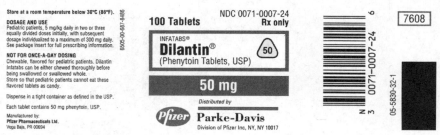

Used with permission from Pfizer, Inc.

Give: _____

8. The client has a medication order for Neurontin (oral solution) 500 milligrams per dose three times a day.

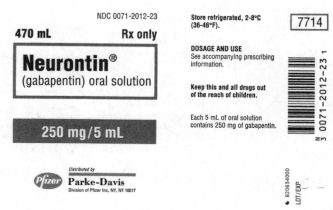

Used with permission from Pfizer, Inc.

Each dose give: _____

9. The nurse is asked to give the client Norvasc 10 milligrams per day.

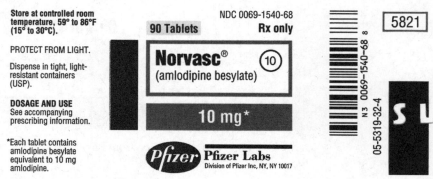

Used with permission from Pfizer, Inc.

Give: _____

10. The physician writes an order for Plendil 7.5 milligrams once a day in the morning.

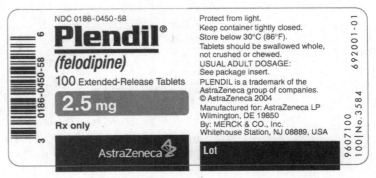

Used with permission from AstraZeneca Pharmaceuticals LP

Give: _____

DOSAGE CALCULATION SELF-TEST

1. The doctor's order is for 20 milligrams. You have 10 milligrams in 5 milliliters. Give _____.

2. Order: 250 milligrams of a drug by mouth. You have scored tables in 100 milligrams dosages. Give _____.

3. Order: pain medication 0.6 gram orally every 4 hours. In the supply are tablets labeled grains v of the pain medication. Give _____.

4. Order: 1.25 milligrams. Have 0.25 milligrams in 5 milliliters. Give _____.

5. Order: Nexium 40 milligrams delayed-release capsules once a day.

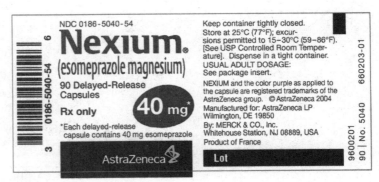

Used with permission from AstraZeneca Pharmaceuticals LP

Give: _____

6. Order: Zocor 80 milligrams per day divided in 3 doses of 20 milligrams, 20 milligrams, and an evening dose of 40 milligrams.

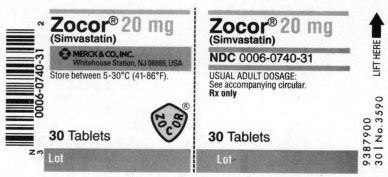

The labels for the products Prinivil, Fosamax, Singulair, Cozaar, Pepcid, Hyzaar, and Zocor are reproduced with the permission of Merck & Co., Inc., copyright owner.

Calculate for the evening dose only. Give: _____

7. Order: Prinivil 15 milligrams once daily.

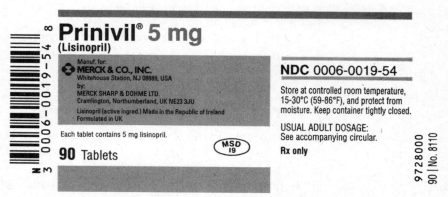

The labels for the products Prinivil, Fosamax, Singulair, Cozaar, Pepcid, Hyzaar, and Zocor are reproduced with the permission of Merck & Co., Inc., copyright owner.

Give: _____

8. The physician orders Cardura 1 milligrams once daily at bedtime.

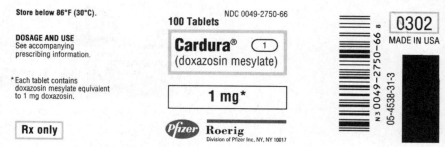

Used with permission from Pfizer, Inc.

Give: _____

9. The doctor orders 200 milligrams of a drug by mouth every 4 hours. The vial contains 125 milligrams in 5 milliliter. Give _____ milliliters.

10. Order: grains iii
    Have: 60 milligram tablets
    Give: _____

11. Order: 50 milligrams orally
    Have: 12.5 milligrams in each 5 milliliters
    Give: _____

12. Order: grain $\dfrac{1}{150}$
    Have: 200 micrograms per tablet
    Give: _____

13. Order: grains v orally
    Have: 0.15 grains per tablet
    Give: _____

14. Dr. Brown orders 0.2 grams of zidovudine in tablets every 4 hours for an HIV patient. The pharmacy carries this medication in 100 milligram tablets. How many tablets will the patient receive? _____

15. The nurse has 15 milligram tablets in her medicine cabinet. Dr. Smith orders 30 milligrams of phenobarbital. She will give _____.

Unit 12

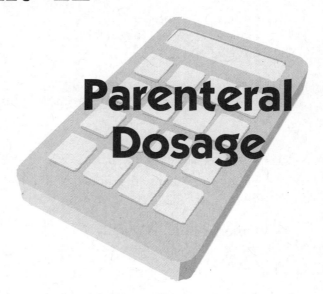

Parenteral Dosage

Parenteral medications are not taken orally. These medications may in the form of injections, inhalants, patches, or suppositories. The common parenteral routes are

Route	Abbreviation	Entry point
intradermal	ID	between the layers of skin
intramuscular	IM	into a muscle
intravenous	IV	into a vein
subcutaneous	sub-Q	under the skin

Injections are mixtures of pure drug dissolved in an appropriate liquid. The dosage or solution strength will be provided on the medication label. The dosage strength will be given in milligrams per milliliter as a ratio or as a percent. It is important to remember that parenteral doses are calculated based on the amount of drug contained in a specific volume of solution. Parenteral dosages are prescribed in grams (g), milligrams (mg), milliequivalent (mEq), or in units (U).

Example of dosage	Given form	Dosage interpretation
Neurontin 250 milligrams / 5 milliliter	milligram per milliliter	5 milliliters contains 250 milligrams of Neurontin
Epinephrine 1:1000	ratio	1000 milliliters contains 1 gram of Epinephrine
Lidocaine 2.5%	percent	100 milliliters contains 2.5 grams of Lidocaine

> ### Review Tip
>
> Ratios such as 2:500 convert to 2 grams in 500 milliliters. Note: No unit of measure is given, so it is critical to remember that in ratios on medication labels the ratio is grams (dry weight) or milliliters (volume) to milliliters.
>
> Thus, 1:1000 translates to 1 gram in 1000 milliliters of solution.
>
> Percents such as 14% convert to 14 grams (or milliliters) in 100 milliliters. The units of measure are also not given, so when a drug label reads 4% that translates to 4 grams or milliliters to 100 milliliter.

Syringes administer parenteral medications. Common syringes are the 3 cubic centimeter per milliliter syringe, the 1 cubic centimeter per milliliter syringe, which is also called the tuberculin syringe, and the insulin syringe, which come in various sizes. The dilution of insulin is such that 1 milliliter of insulin fluid has 100 standard units of insulin. Note that cubic centimeter and milliliter are equal; both measures are used. There are other syringe sizes; however, the following are the most common syringes used for parenteral dosages.

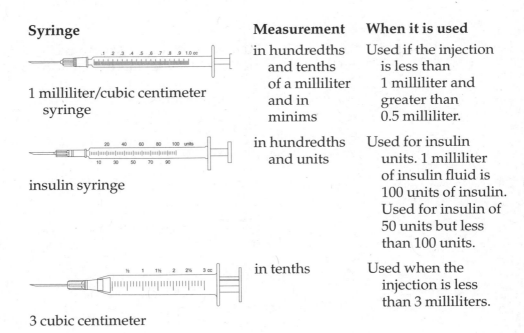

Syringe	Measurement	When it is used
1 milliliter/cubic centimeter syringe	in hundredths and tenths of a milliliter and in minims	Used if the injection is less than 1 milliliter and greater than 0.5 milliliter.
insulin syringe	in hundredths and units	Used for insulin units. 1 milliliter of insulin fluid is 100 units of insulin. Used for insulin of 50 units but less than 100 units.
3 cubic centimeter	in tenths	Used when the injection is less than 3 milliliters.

For IM injections, there are guidelines for maximum volumes for injection sites. This is important for accurate dosage calculation and consideration of multiple syringes. Any dosage larger than the recommended amount is usually checked and verified with the physician and the dosage is then divided equally or as close to equal as possible and given in two separate injection sites.

Client	Age	Maximum dose per site
Adult	12+	3 milliliter IM or 1 milliliter deltoid arm
Child	6–12 years	2 milliliter
Child	0–5 years	1 milliliter
Infant	Premature	0.5 milliliter

In addition to the apothecary, metric, and household measures, health care has two other units of measure commonly used in client medication orders.

Medications are also prescribed in milliequivalents (mEq) and units (U). One milliequivalent equals one-thousandth ($^1/_{1000}$). Sodium, potassium, sodium bicarbonate, and potassium chloride are commonly prescribed in milliequivalents. A unit is a standardized amount needed to produce a certain desired effect of a medication. Units are used to prescribe medications such as heparin, insulin, and penicillin. No conversions are used because these medications are prescribed in milliequivalents per milliliter (mEq/mL) or units per milliliter (U/mL) and the labeling matches these measures.

To calculate the dosage, there are several means of getting to the correct dose. One may use the dosage formula, ratio and proportion, or dimensional analysis. Choose the method that you are most comfortable with and use it consistently. An example of each follows.

Example   The doctor has ordered 500 milligrams of Ampicillin be given. On hand is a vial labeled Ampicillin 250 milligrams in 5 cubic centimeters.

To solve with the dosage formula:

$$\frac{\text{ordered dosage}}{\text{supply on hand}} \times \text{quantity} = \text{dosage to be given}$$

Set up

$$\frac{500 \text{ milligrams}}{250 \text{ milligrams}} \times 5 \text{ cubic centimeters} = \text{dosage to be given}$$

Solve

$$\frac{500 \text{ milligrams}}{250 \text{ milligrams}} \times 5 \text{ cubic centimeters} = \frac{2}{1} \times 5 \text{ cubic centimeters}$$

$$= 10 \text{ cubic centimeters}$$

To solve with ratio and proportion:

Set up

500 milligrams : ? cubic centimeters :: 250 milligrams : 5 cubic centimeters

Solve

a. $\dfrac{500 \text{ milligrams}}{? \text{ cubic centimeters}} = \dfrac{250 \text{ milligrams}}{5 \text{ cubic centimeters}} =$

b. $500 \times 5 = 2500$

c. $\dfrac{2500}{250} = 10 \text{ cubic centimeters}$

To solve with dimensional analysis:

a. Place the unknown unit on the left side of the equation (what you are solving)

$$? \text{ cubic centimeter} =$$

b. The dosage unit of measure is 5 cubic centimeters. The dose on hand is 250 milligrams. Use this known information to form the first factor.

$$? \text{ cubic centimeters} = \dfrac{5 \text{ cubic centimeters}}{250 \text{ milligrams}}$$

c. The physician has ordered 500 milligrams. Place the 500 milligrams over 1 to form the second factor of the equation.

$$? \text{ cubic centimeters} = \dfrac{5 \text{ cubic centimeters}}{250 \text{ milligrams}} \times \dfrac{500 \text{ milligrams}}{1}$$

d. Cancel like units and solve.

$$? \text{ cubic centimeters} = \dfrac{5 \text{ cubic centimeters}}{250 \text{ milligrams}} \times \dfrac{500 \text{ milligrams}}{1} \rightarrow \dfrac{5}{1} \times \dfrac{2}{1}$$

$$= 10 \text{ cubic centimeters}$$

Practice   Solve the following parenteral dosages. Round to the nearest tenth.

1. Order: Ephedrine sulfate 12.5 milligrams subcutaneously
   Have: Vial labeled ephedrine sulfate 25 milligrams per milliliter
   Give: _____

2. Order: Diazepam 2 milligram IM
   Have: Vial labeled Diazepam 5 milligrams per milliliter
   Give: _____ Shade the syringe.

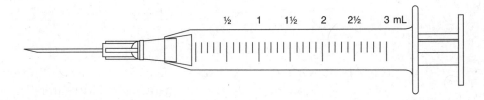

3. Order: Kefzol 500 milligram IM every 6 hours
   Have: Label reads Kefzol 225 milligrams per milliliter
   Give: _____

4. Order: Colchicine IV 0.5 milligram
   Have: Vial labeled colchicine IV 500 micrograms per milliliter
   Give: _____

5. Order: Amitriptyline 25 milligrams IM
   Have: Vial labeled amitriptyline 10 milligrams per milliliter
   Give: _____ Shade the syringe.

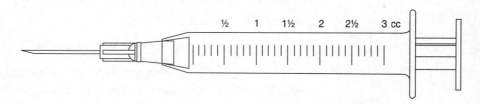

6. Order: Add to IV: Bretylium 500 milligrams
   Have: Bretylium 50 milligrams per milliliter
   Give: _____

7. Order: Furosemide 20 milligrams IV
   Have: Furosemide 10 milligrams per milliliter
   Give: _____

8. Order: Nafcillin 500 milligrams IM
   Have: When 3.4 milliliters of diluent is added to 1 gram vial,
              250 milligrams = 1 milliliter
   Give: _____ Shade the syringe.

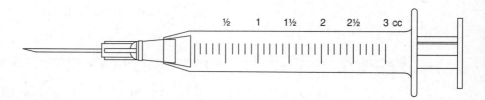

9. Order: Phenergen 25 milligrams
   Have: Phenergen 50 milligrams per milliliter
   Give: _____ Shade the syringe.

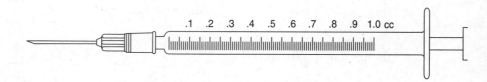

10. Order: As pre-op, give morphine 8 milligrams
    Have: Morphine grain $\frac{1}{6}$ in 2 milliliters
    Give: _____

Additional Practice

Solve the following Parenteral dosages. Round to the nearest tenth.

1. The physician orders heparin 5000 units. The heparin label reads 10,000 units per milliliter.
   Give _____

2. Give penicillin G 100,000 units form a vial labeled 1,000,000 units in 5 milliliter.
   Give _____

3. The physician has ordered Decadron 3 milligrams from a vial labeled 4 milligrams per milliliter.
   Give _____ Shade the syringe.

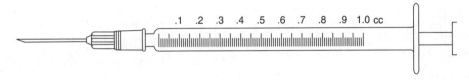

4. Give heparin 15,000 units IV. The vial is labeled heparin 1000 units per milliliter.
   Give _____

5. Give lidocaine 200 milligrams IM stat from a vial labeled lidocaine 10%.
   Give _____

6. The physician has ordered lanoxin 125 micrograms IM daily. The drug label reads 250 micrograms (25 milligrams) per milliliter.
   Give _____

7. The client is in pain. The physician's order is for Demerol 75 milligrams every 4 hours IM as needed for pain. The Demerol label reads 100 milligrams in 2 milliliter.
   Give _____ Shade the syringe.

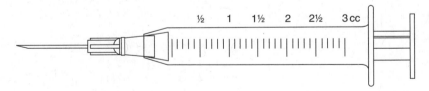

8. The drug order reads, give Prostigmin 0.5 milligram IM stat. The drug label reads, Prostigmin 1:2000 solution.
   Give _____

9. The physician has ordered phenylephrine 2.5 milligrams sub-Q for the client. The drug label on the vial reads 10 milligrams per milliliter.
   Give _____

10. Dr. Smith has ordered morphine sulfate grain $\frac{1}{12}$. The morphine sulfate vial is labeled 10 milligrams per milliliter.
    Give _____

PARENTERAL DOSAGE SELF-TEST

1. The physician orders Loxitane 30 milligrams IM every 12 hours. The Loxitane label reads 50 milligrams per milliliter.
   Give _____ Shade the syringe.

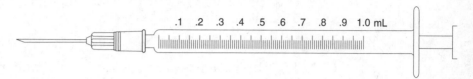

2. Give Dilaudid 0.5 milligram IM from a vial that is labeled 2 milligrams per milliliter.
   Give _____

3. Order: Atropine 0.6 milligrams IV
   Have: Atropine 0.8 milligram per milliliter
   Give: _____

4. The physician has ordered calcitonin 100 units IM for the client. The calcitonin vial reads 400 units in 2 milliliters.
   Give_____ Shade the syringe.

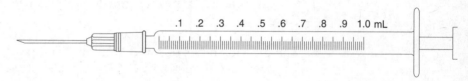

5. The physician has ordered adrenalin 0.5 milligram sub-Q stat. The adrenalin label reads 1:1000 solution.
   Give _____

6. Order: Cefazolin Sodium 250 milligrams IM every 8 hours
   Have: Cefazolin Sodium 500 milligrams in 5 cubic centimeters
   Give: _____ Shade the syringe.

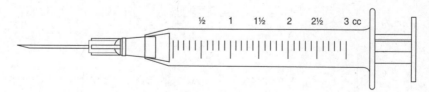

7. The physician has ordered magnesium sulfate 550 milligrams stat. The magnesium sulfate vial is labeled 20% solution.
   Give _____

8. Give Butorphanol 0.5 milligrams IV for the client every 3 to 4 hours. The Butorphanol drug label reads 2 milligrams per milliliter.
   Give _____

9. The physician orders Imitrex 4 milligrams sub-Q as needed for headache every 4 to 6 hours for the client. The Imitrex drug label on the vial reads 12 milligrams per milliliter.
Give _____ Shade the syringe.

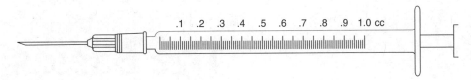

10. Order: Zemplar 3 micrograms IM
    Have: Zemplar 5 micrograms per milliliter
    Give: _____ Shade the syringe.

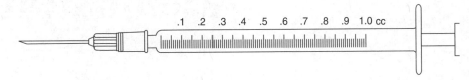

11. The physician has ordered Levsin 1 milligram IM four times a day for the client. The drug label on the vial reads 0.5 milligram hyoscyamine sulfate injection USP per milliliter of water.
Give _____

12. Order: Lidocaine 25 milligrams sub-Q
    Have: Lidocaine 5% solution
    Give: _____

13. The physician has ordered heparin 25,000 units IV from a vial that reads heparin 1000 units per milliliter.
Give _____

14. Order: Zantac 35 milligrams IM stat
    Have: Zantac 25 milligrams per milliliter
    Give: _____ Shade the syringe.

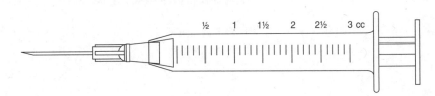

15. The physician has ordered naloxone hydrochloride 0.01 milligram IV from a vial labeled 0.02 milligram per milliliter. The nurse should administer _____

Unit 13

The Basics of Intravenous Fluid Administration

Intravenous (IV) fluids and medications are solutions that are placed directly into the bloodstream via a vein. This is called infusion. Intravenous medications and solutions have a very quick effect. Intravenous medications are used for critical care situations. Moderate to large doses of fluids or medications are given this way. An IV medication may be prepared by a physician, nurse, pharmacist, or a pharmacy technician. IV solutions are also used to maintain and to replace fluids, to keep a vein open for further treatment, and to provide therapy.

The following are the common abbreviations used in IV administration:

Term	Abbreviation
Intravenous	IV
Piggy-back	PB
Drop/drops	gtt/gtts
Hour	hr
Minutes	min
Drops per minute	gtts/min
Drops per milliliter	gtts/mL
Milliliters per hour	mL/hr
Water	H_2O, W

5% dextrose water	D_5W
10% dextrose water	$D_{10}W$
Normal saline (0.9%)	NS
One half normal saline (0.45%)	$\frac{1}{2}$ NS
Ringer's lactate solution	RL
Lactated Ringer's solution	LR

An IV infusion set is used to administer fluids and medications. An IV infusion set has several parts: a sealed plastic bag or a bottle, a drip chamber, tubing, and a needle or catheter at the insertion site into the patient. Infusion or flow rates are adjusted to the desired drops per minute by a clamp on the tubing. The infusion administration set tracks the number of drops being delivered. It should be noted that the larger the tubing the larger the drop.

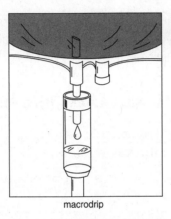 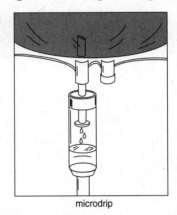

macrodrip   microdrip

There are both manual and electronic infusion pumps in use today. The electronic infusion pumps require less computation on the part of the nurse as these machines have a controller that measures the drops or volume for a preset flow rate. The nurse monitors the equipment and the client to ensure proper and safe use. For manual IV sets, the flow rate is calculated in drops per minute (gtts/min). To calculate this, one must know the administration set drop factor. Macrodrip tubing administers a larger drop and may be used for 10 drops per milliliter, 15 drops per milliliter, or 20 drops per milliliter. Microdrip tubing administers 60 drops per milliliter.

Nurses often need to use information on drug orders to calculate the IV infusion rates. The drug order will include the type of fluid, the amount of fluid, and the number of hours that the fluid is to be infused. IV administration sets are predetermined by the manufacturer to deliver a certain number of drops per minute per milliliter of fluid that is given. Nurses, if unfamiliar with the type of administration set, should read the label on the machine. In general, the following drip rates are used:

Microdrip administration	60 drops per milliliter
Standard administration/macrodrip administration	10, 15, 20 drops per milliliter
Blood administration	10 drops per milliliter

These are called *drop factors.* The drop factor is the number of drops contained in 1 milliliter. Large volumes of fluid require a macrodrip administration. Macrodrip sets run 125 milliliters per hour or more, whereas microdrip sets run 50 milliliter per hour or less. These rates are often specified by the facility to ensure proper drug administration. Nurses are responsible for ensuring that the IV flow is regular. They monitor flow rate and ensure needle placement, condition of the vein, and patient safety and comfort.

Health care professionals see flow rates expressed in a variety of ways. You will need to solve these calculations using the information that is presented in each problem, which will require the application of literal equations

$$\text{Rate(flow rate)} = \frac{\text{Volume}}{\text{Time}} \rightarrow R = \frac{V}{t}$$

> Review:
> Solve literal equations by performing the inverse operations (V, t, or R) until you have solved the equation.

To Calculate IV Infusion Rates with a Formula

$$\frac{\text{Amount of fluid in milliliters (mL)}}{\text{Total time of infusion in minutes}} \times \text{Administration set drop factor}$$

$$= \text{Drops per minute}$$

> Note: A shortcut can be used to handle the hours to minutes conversion. Then, cancellation is used to reduce the amount of calculation used.

Example   To administer 500 milliliters of IV fluid over 12 hours using a microdrip administration set, how many drops per minute would the nurse administer? (Hint: Microdrip has a drop factor of 60 drops per minute.)
Set up

$$\frac{500 \text{ milliliter}}{12 \text{ hours} \times 60 \text{ minutes}} \times 60 \text{ drop factor} = \underline{\qquad} \text{ drops per minute}$$

Working through the formula:

Step 1. Do not multiply 12×60 because cross cancellation will reduce or eliminate the 60.

$$\frac{500 \text{ milliliter}}{12 \times \cancel{60}} \times \cancel{60} = \underline{\qquad} \text{ drops per minute}$$

$$500 \div 12 = 41.6666$$

The answer is 42 drops per minute

> Remember: Drops must be rounded up or down to ensure a whole number of drops. There are no partial drops. Thus, drops per minute and drops per hour will be whole numbers.

To calculate IV infusion rates with dimensional analysis

To administer 500 milliliter of IV fluid over 12 hours using a microdrip administration set, how many drops per minute would the nurse administer? (Hint: Microdrip has a drop factor of 60 drops per minute.)

a. Set up the unknown quantity on one side of the equation. We are solving drops per minute.

$$z \text{ drops per minute} =$$

b. The first factor is the total amount to be administered in milliliters over the time in hours.

$$z \text{ drops per minute} = \frac{500 \text{ milliliters}}{12 \text{ hours}}$$

c. The second factor is the hours to minutes conversion. This is multiplied by the first factor.

$$z \text{ drops per minute} = \frac{500 \text{ milliliters}}{12 \text{ hours}} \times \frac{1 \text{ hour}}{60 \text{ minutes}}$$

d. Multiply this by the drop factor.

$$z \text{ drops per minute} = \frac{500 \text{ milliliters}}{12 \text{ hours}} \times \frac{1 \text{ hour}}{60 \text{ minutes}} \times \frac{60 \text{ drop}}{1 \text{ milliliter}}$$

e. Cancel like units and then solve. (Convert values to like units where appropriate.)

$$z \text{ drops per minute} = \frac{500 \text{ milliliters}}{12 \text{ hours}} \times \frac{1 \text{ hour}}{60 \text{ minutes}} \times \frac{60 \text{ drop}}{1 \text{ milliliter}}$$

$$z \text{ drops per minute} = 500 \div 12 = 41.6666$$

The answer is 42 drops per minute

Practice   Use one of the above methods to complete the following calculations of IV flow rates. Round your answers to the nearest whole number.

	Amount of fluid in milliliters	Time in hours	IV set drop factor	Drops per minute
1	300	3	60	_____
2	1000	12	60	_____
3	125	3	10	_____
4	350	4	60	_____
5	2500	24	60	_____
6	450	8	20	_____
7	24	1	60	_____
8	1000	24	15	_____
9	600	12	20	_____
10	250	8	60	_____
11	1600	12	60	_____
12	48	3	15	_____
13	1800	18	15	_____
14	1500	12	60	_____
15	150	24	60	_____
16	675	8	60	_____
17	320	5	15	_____
18	200	$1\frac{1}{2}$	20	_____
19	1400	8	15	_____
20	900	12	60	_____

Additional Practice

Find the drops per minute for each of the following problems.

1. The physician has ordered D_5W 1500 milliliters in 12 hours using a 15 drops per milliliter infusion rate. Infuse at _____ drops per minute.

2. The registered nurse is to infuse the 1 unit of whole plasma (500 milliliters) over 4 hours using a blood administration rate of 10 drops per milliliter. Infuse at _____ drops per minute.

3. The nurse reads the physician's order for 1000 milliliters of $D_5 \frac{1}{4}$ NS over 12 hours at 15 drops per milliliters. Infuse at _____.

4. Infuse 325 milliliters $D_5 \frac{1}{2}$ NS over 4 hours. Use 60 drops per milliliter. Infuse at _____.

5. The nurse receives a physician's order for 300 milliliters plasma over 8 hours at 10 drops per milliliter. Infuse at _____.

6. Infuse 1200 milliliters D_5 LR over 24 hours at 15 drops per milliliter. Infuse at _____.

7. The nurse is asked to infuse D_5 $\frac{1}{3}$ NS 500 milliliters over 4 hours using microdrip tubing. Infuse at _____.

8. The physician prescribes Ionosol MB 750 milliliters over 12 hours using microdrip tubing. Infuse at _____.

9. The registered nurse received client Howard's medication order for 250 milliliters of packed red cells over 4 hours using a blood administration rate of 10 drops per milliliter. Infuse at _____.

10. An order reads D_5W 1000 milliliters infused over 24 hours at 20 drops per milliliter. Infuse at _____.

These types of calculations are straightforward when all the parts of the calculation are given. However, there are instances when one must calculate the missing part of the problem. In this case, a modified setup may be required. The possible unknowns may be flow rate, infusion time, and total volume.

To find the mL/hr, use this basic formula:

$$\frac{V}{t} = F$$

> V = volume in milliliters
>
> t = time in hours
>
> F = flow rate in milliliter per hour to nearest whole number

Example   The doctor has prescribed 750 milligrams of Ampicillin in 125 milliliters NS to infuse over 45 minutes. What is the milliliter per hour infusion rate?

To solve with the formula method

Set up

$$\frac{V}{t} = F$$

> $$\frac{1 \text{ hour}}{60 \text{ minutes}} = \frac{x \text{ hour}}{45 \text{ minutes}} \rightarrow 1 \times 45 = 45$$
>
> Then $\rightarrow 45 \div 60 = 0.75$ hour

$$\frac{125 \text{ milliliters}}{45 \text{ minutes}} \rightarrow 45 \text{ minutes is } \frac{45}{60} \text{ or } 0.75 \text{ hour}$$

Solve

$$\frac{125 \text{ milliliters}}{0.75 \text{ hour}} = 166.666 \text{ milliliters per hour}$$

> Remember: Drops are rounded to the nearest whole number.

The answer is 167 milliliters per hour

To solve using dimensional analysis

a. The unknown to be solved is the flow rate is placed on the left of the equal to that sign.

$$? \text{ milliliters per hour} =$$

b. The first factor is $V/_t$ and it is placed in the equation.

$$? \text{ milliliters per hour} = \frac{125 \text{ milliliters}}{45 \text{ minutes}}$$

c. Multiply the first factor by the second factor, which is the conversion of minutes to parts of an hour.

$$? \text{ milliliters per hour} = \frac{125 \text{ milliliters}}{45 \text{ minutes}} \times \frac{60 \text{ minutes}}{1 \text{ hour}}$$

(Note: this step may not be necessary if the problem uses hours instead of minutes.)

d. Cancel like units of measure and solve.

$$? \text{ milliliters per hour} = \frac{125 \text{ milliliters}}{45 \text{ minutes}} \times \frac{60 \text{ minutes}}{1 \text{ hour}} \rightarrow \frac{7500}{45}$$

$$= 166.66 \text{ milliliters per hour}$$
$$\text{or } 167 \text{ milliliters per hour}$$

Practice   Choose a method and calculate these problems to find _____ milliliters per hour.

1. 1 liter of D_5W IV to infuse in 12 hours by infusion pump. Infuse at _____ milliliters per hour.

2. Infuse 50 milliliters of antibiotic in D_5W in 30 minutes. Infuse at _____ milliliters per hour.

3. The nurse is asked to infuse 150 milliliters NS IV PB in 30 minutes. Infuse at _____ milliliters per hour.

4. Infuse 1800 milliliters NS IV in 24 hours. Infuse at _____ milliliters per hour.

5. Infuse 2000 milliliters D_5W IV in 18 hours. Infuse at _____ milliliters per hour.

6. Infuse 650 milliliters D_5 0.45% NaCl IV for 5 hours. Infuse at _____ milliliters per hour.

7. The physician orders 1000 milliliters $D_{10}W$ to infuse over 8 hours. Infuse at _____ milliliters per hour.

8. The physician's order is for D_5NS 1200 milliliters to infuse over 24 hours. Infuse at _____ milliliters per hour.

9. The nurse receives an order for 600 milliliters Normosol R over 8 hours. Infuse at _____ milliliters per hour.

10. Infuse 1400 milliliters of medication over 6 hours. Infuse at _____ milliliters per hour.

Sometimes the infusion time in hours (a specific duration) is not given. The following formula will help solve the problem.

$$t = \frac{V}{F}$$

> t = specific time in hours
> V = volume in milliliters (mL)
> F = flow rate in milliliters per hour

Example   The physician orders $D_5 \frac{1}{2} NS$ 1000 milliliters at 175 milliliters per hour.

To solve using the formula method:

Set up

$$t = \frac{V}{F} \rightarrow t = \frac{1000 \text{ milliliters}}{175 \text{ milliliters per hour}}$$

Solve

$$t = \frac{1000 \text{ milliliters}}{175 \text{ milliliters per hour}} \rightarrow 1000 \div 175$$

$$= 5.71428 \text{ hours for infusing 1000 milliliters}$$

Round to the nearest hundredth—5.71 hours. Note the decimal portion of the answer must be in minutes.

To convert the decimal number to hours and minutes

a. Separate the whole number from decimal number—5 hours and 0.71

b. Multiply the decimal number 0.71 × 60 minutes.

0.71 × 60 = 42.6 minutes. Round to the nearest minute—43 minutes

c. Place the hours and minutes together.

5 hours 43 minutes

The answer is 5 hours 43 minutes.

To solve using dimensional analysis

a. The unknown is the unit of time (t) in hours (h). Place on the left of the equation.

$$t\, h =$$

b. Place the first factor which is the total number of milliliters to be infused over one.

$$t\, h = \frac{1000 \text{ milliliters}}{1}$$

c. Then multiply the first factor by the inverse of the flow rate.

$$t\, h = \frac{1000 \text{ milliliters}}{1} \times \frac{1 \text{ hour}}{175 \text{ milliliters}}$$

d. Cancel like units and then solve.

$$t\, h = \frac{1000}{175} \rightarrow 5.71428$$

e. To convert the decimal number to hours and minutes

Step 1: Separate the whole number from decimal number—5 hours and 0.71.

Step 2: Multiply the decimal number—0.71 × 60 minutes.

0.71 × 60 = 42.6 minutes. Round to the nearest minute—43 minutes.

Step 3: Place the hours and minutes together.

5 hours 43 minutes

Practice   Solve the following by calculating the infusion times in hours.

1. The nurse receives an order that reads: 500 milliliters D_5W IV at 50 milliliters per hour. Infuse for _____.

2. A baby is to receive 300 milliliters D_5NS at 25 milliliters per hour. Infuse for _____.

3. Infuse 2000 milliliters at 125 milliliters per hour. Infuse for _____.

4. The patient is to receive LR 1000 milliliters at 140 milliliters per hour. Infuse for _____.

5. A nurse is requested to infuse 600 milliliters Normosol R at 125 milliliters per hour. Infuse for _____.

6. Ordered: 1000 milliliters NS at 200 milliliters per hour. What is the total time of infusion? _____.

7. Ordered: 650 milliliters D_5W at 83 milliliters per hour. What is the total time of infusion? _____.

8. Ordered: 800 milliliters NS at 75 milliliters per hour. What is the total time of infusion? _____.

9. Ordered: 750 milliliters RL at 83 milliliters per hour. What is the total time of infusion? _____.

10. Ordered: 1800 milliliters 0.45% NS at 75 milliliters per hour. What is the total time of infusion? _____.

Sometimes the total volume of fluid to be infused must be calculated.
   To calculate how much fluid will be infused, one may use a formula or dimensional analysis:

$$V = t \times F$$

> V = volume in milliliters (mL)
> t = time in hours
> F = flow rate in milliliters per hour

Example   What is the total volume infused in 8 hours if the infusion rate is 65 milliliters per hour?

To solve with the formula

$V = t \times F$ where t = 5 hours and F = 65 milliliters per hour

5 hours $\times$ 65 milliliters per hour = 325 milliliters in total volume

To solve with dimensional analysis

a. Determine the unit of measure for the unknown volume and place it on the left side of the equation.

$$V \text{ milliliter} =$$

b. The first factor is the length of time over one.

$$V \text{ milliliter} = \frac{5 \text{ hours}}{1}$$

c. Multiply the first factor by the flow rate, which is the second factor.

$$V \text{ milliliter} = \frac{5 \text{ hours}}{1} \times \frac{65 \text{ milliliters}}{1 \text{ hour}}$$

d. Cancel like units and solve.

$$V \text{ milliliter} = \frac{5 \text{ hours}}{1} \times \frac{65 \text{ milliliters}}{1 \text{ hour}} \rightarrow \frac{5 \times 65}{1}$$

$$= 325 \text{ milliliters to be infused in 5 hours}$$

Practice   Solve the total volume to be infused.

1. Ordered: D_5 $\frac{1}{2}$ NS IV at 125 milliliters per hour for 12 hours. What is the total volume infused? _____

2. Ordered: Penicillin IV over 4 hours at a rate of 75 milliliters per hour. What is the total volume infused? _____

3. The nurse will administer an IV solution at 83 milliliters per hour for 6 hours. What is the total volume infused? _____

4. The patient will receive an IV therapy that runs at 120 milliliters per hour for 12 hours. What is the total volume infused? _____

5. The physician has ordered a therapeutic IV solution at 31 milliliters per hour for 18 hours. What is the total volume infused? _____

6. The nurse will administer $\frac{1}{2}$ NS IV at 50 milliliters per hour for 6 hours. What is the total volume infused? _____

7. Ordered: D_5 RL IV at 67 milliliters per hour for 4 hours. What is the total volume infused? _____

8. The physician has ordered an antibiotic IV solution at 125 milliliters per hour for a total of 12 hours. What is the total volume infused? _____

9. Ordered: 100 milliliters of 0.45% NS IV for 4 hours. What is the total volume infused? _____

10. The nurse will prepare to administer $D_{10}W$ IV at 33 milliliters per hour for 24 hours. What is the total volume infused? _____

THE BASICS OF INTRAVENOUS FLUID ADMINISTRATION SELF-TEST

Calculate the drops per minute for each of the following:

	Total volume for infusion in milliliters	Time in hours	Drop factor	Answer (drops per minute)
1.	500	8	15	_____
2.	250	6	20	_____
3.	1500	12	60	_____
4.	125	4	10	_____
5.	750	8	60	_____

Find milliliters per hour rate for each of the following:

	Total volume in milliliters	Total infusion time	Answer (milliliter per hour)
6.	1200	6 hours	_____
7.	750	12 hours	_____
8.	250	4 hours	_____
9.	1800	24 hours	_____
10.	100	30 minutes	_____

Calculate the total infusion time for each of the following:

	Total volume in milliliters	Infusion rate milliliters per hour	Answer (Time in hours)
11.	500	125	_____
12.	650	133	_____
13.	1,200	60	_____
14.	1,000	100	_____
15.	250	83	_____

Find the total volume to be infused for each of the following:

	Flow rate in milliliters per hour	Time in hours	Total volume in milliliters
16.	135	6	_____
17.	83	8	_____
18.	25	3	_____
19.	125	12	_____
20.	65	$2\frac{1}{2}$	_____

Unit 14

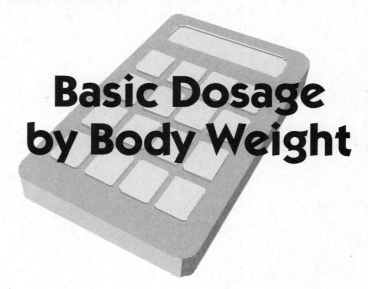

Basic Dosage by Body Weight

Special population drug orders such as pediatric and geriatric medications are often calculated based on weight. These drug orders will state a medication amount per patient weight for a specific time. For example, the drug order reads Methotrexate sodium IV 2.5 milligrams per kilogram every 14 days. The nurse will calculate the dose by multiplying 2.5 milligrams by the patient's weight in kilograms to compute the intravenous dose to be given every 14 days.

Converting a patient's weight to kilogram requires knowledge of basic math and the metric system. The first step is to convert the weight from pounds and ounces into kilograms.

Example The client weighs 32 pounds. What is his weight in kilograms?

To convert pounds to kilograms with a formula
Set up

$$\frac{1 \text{ kilogram}}{2.2 \text{ pounds}} = \frac{? \text{ kilograms}}{32 \text{ pounds}}$$

Solve

a. 1 kilogram $\times$ 32 = 32

b. $\frac{32}{2.2}$ = 14.5454545

c. Round to the nearest hundredth.

The answer is 14.55 kilograms.

> Note: For calculating accurate dosages, the kilogram weight is rounded to the nearest hundredth for dosage by weight calculations.

To convert pounds to kilograms with dimensional analysis

The client weighs 32 pounds. What is his weight in kilograms?

a. Place the unknown weight on the left side of the equation.

$$? \text{ kilograms} =$$

b. Then the first factor is the conversion rate.

$$? \text{ kilograms} = \frac{1 \text{ kilogram}}{2.2 \text{ pounds}}$$

c. Multiply the first factor by the weight in pounds over 1.

$$? \text{ kilograms} = \frac{1 \text{ kilogram}}{2.2 \text{ pounds}} \times \frac{32 \text{ pounds}}{1} =$$

d. Cancel like units and solve.

$$? \text{ kilograms} = \frac{1 \text{ kilogram}}{2.2 \text{ pounds}} \times \frac{32 \text{ pounds}}{1} \rightarrow \frac{32}{2.2} = 14.54545$$

e. Round to the nearest hunderedth.

The answer is 14.55 kilograms.

Practice   Convert the weight in pounds to weight in kilograms. Round to the nearest hundredth.

	Weight in pounds	Weight in kilograms
1.	14	_____
2.	55	_____
3.	27	_____
4.	98	_____
5.	40	_____
6.	110	_____
7.	16	_____
8.	8	_____
9.	30	_____
10.	105	_____

When a pound weight includes ounces, use the same method but first convert the ounces to a decimal.

For example, Convert 14 pounds 4 ounces to kilograms.

$$14 \text{ pounds } 4 \text{ ounces } = 14\frac{4}{16}$$

$$= 14\frac{1}{4} \text{ or } 14.25 \text{ pounds.}$$

> Remember that 1 pound has 16 ounces.

Convert 25 pounds 10 ounces to kilograms.
Separate the ounces and place them in fraction form over 16.
25 pounds and $^{10}/_{16}$. When $^{10}/_{16}$ is divided and made into a decimal the result is 0.625.

Thus, the pound weight becomes 25.625 and is then ready to convert with either method of conversion. Once the math is completed, round the kilogram to the nearest hundredth.

Practice   Convert the pounds to kilograms.

	Weight in pounds and ounces	Decimal number to be converted to kilograms	Kilograms
1.	14 pounds 8 ounces	_____	_____
2.	22 pounds 5 ounces	_____	_____
3.	16 pounds 4 ounces	_____	_____
4.	31 pounds 6 ounces	_____	_____
5.	42 pounds 2 ounces	_____	_____
6.	9 pounds 8 ounces	_____	_____
7.	12 pounds 12 ounces	_____	_____
8.	109 pounds 8 ounces	_____	_____
9.	124 pounds 14 ounces	_____	_____
10.	7 pounds 10 ounces	_____	_____

Once the weight is converted from pounds to kilograms, then the next step is to calculate the dosage by multiplying the dose ordered by the weight in kilograms.

Example   The nurse receives a medication order for a child: Vancomycin hydrochloride 40 milligrams per kilogram per day in four divided doses for 10 days, not to exceed 2 grams a day. The child weighs 34 pounds 6 ounces. What is the total daily dose? What is the individual dose?

To solve with the proportional method

1. Convert 34 pounds 6 ounces to kilograms

   a. 34 pounds and $^{6}/_{16}$ → 6 ÷ 16 = 0.375 or 0.38

      34.38 pounds

b. Set up

$$\frac{1 \text{ kilogram}}{2.2 \text{ pounds}} = \frac{? \text{ kilograms}}{34.38 \text{ pounds}}$$

c. Solve

$$1 \times 34.38 = 34.38$$

$$34.38 \div 2.2 = 15.6272 \text{ or } 15.63 \text{ kilograms}$$

2. Carefully reread the math problem
40 milligrams per kilogram per day in four divided doses for 10 days

Set up

$$40 \times 15.63 =$$

Solve

$40 \times 15.63 = 625.2$ milligrams per day in four divided doses for 10 days

625.2 divided into four doses $(625.2 \div 4 = 156.3)$

> Daily dosage is 625.2 milligrams
>
> Individual dose every 6 hours(four times a day) is 156.3 milligrams.

Example   The nurse receives a medication order for a child: Vancomycin hydrochloride 40 milligrams per kilogram per day in four divided doses for 10 days, not to exceed 2 grams a day. The child weighs 34 pounds 6 ounces. What is the total daily dose? What is the individual dose?

To solve with dimensional analysis

1. Convert the 34 pounds 6 ounces to kilograms

$$34 \text{ pounds and } ^6\!/_{16} \rightarrow 6 \div 16 = 0.375 \text{ or } 0.38$$

$$34.38 \text{ pounds}$$

a. Place the unknown on the left side of the equation and the conversion as the first factor which is multiplied by the decimal weight.

$$? \text{ kilograms} = \frac{1 \text{ kilogram}}{2.2 \text{ pounds}} \times 34.38 \text{ pounds}$$

b. Cancel like units and solve

$$? \text{ kilograms} = \frac{34.38}{2.2} = 15.63 \text{ kilograms}$$

2. Calculate the dosage

    a. Set up the unknown on the left side of the equation.

$$? \text{ milligrams per day} =$$

    b. Add the first factor which from the problem: 40 milligrams per kilogram per day

$$? \text{ milligrams per day} = \frac{40 \text{ milligrams per day}}{1 \text{ kilogram}}$$

    c. Multiply the first factor by the weight in kilograms.

$$? \text{ milligrams per day} = \frac{40 \text{ milligrams per day}}{1 \text{ kilogram}} \times 15.63 \text{ kilograms}$$

    d. Cancel like units and solve.

$$? \text{ milligrams per day} = \frac{40 \text{ milligrams per day}}{1 \text{ kilogram}} \times 15.63 \text{ kilograms}$$

$$\rightarrow 40 \text{ milligrams} \times 15.63 = 625.2 \text{ milligrams per day}$$

    e. Solve for the individual dose.

      1. Place the dose per day on the left side of the equation.

$$? \text{ individual dose} =$$

      2. Place the first factor, which is the daily dose over 1 day.

$$? \text{ individual dose} = \frac{625.2 \text{ milligrams}}{1 \text{ day}}$$

      3. Multiply the first factor by the second factor, which is the number of doses or $^{1\,day}/_{4\,doses}$ because 4 doses are to be administered in a day.

$$? \text{ individual dose} = \frac{625.2 \text{ milligrams}}{1 \text{ day}} \times \frac{1 \text{ day}}{4 \text{ doses}} =$$

      4. Cancel like units and solve.

$$? \text{ individual dose} = \frac{625.2 \text{ milligrams}}{1 \text{ day}} \times \frac{1 \text{ day}}{4 \text{ doses}}$$

$$\rightarrow \frac{625.2 \text{ milligrams}}{4 \text{ doses}} = 156.3 \text{ milligrams}$$

The answer is 156.3 milligrams per individual dose.

> **Review**
>
> Pound weights that consist of pound and ounces require that the ounces be converted to a decimal number and rounded to the nearest hundredth before being divided by 2.2 to convert the weight in kilograms.
>
> Remember for these dosages, kilograms are rounded to the nearest hundredth place before calculating the individual and daily doses.

Practice   Solve the dosage by weight conversion problems.

1. Weight: 8 pounds 10 ounces
   Recommended dose from drug label: 15 milligrams per kilogram over 24 hours
   What is the weight in kilograms? _____
   What is the daily dose? _____

2. Weight: 12 pounds 4 ounces
   Recommended dose from drug label: 100 milligrams per kilogram every 12 hours
   What is the weight in kilograms? _____
   What is the individual dose? _____

3. Weight: 18 pounds
   Recommended dose from drug label: 0.25 milliliter per kilogram per dose
   What is the weight in kilograms? _____
   What is the individual dose? Round to the nearest whole number.
   _____

4. Weight: 40 pounds 6 ounces
   Ordered dose: Aspirin 300 milligrams not to exceed 1200 milligrams a day.
   Recommended dose from drug label: 65 milligrams per kilogram over 24 hours
   Does the doctor's order fit within the recommended safe guidelines of not exceeding 1200 milligrams per day? _____ What is the daily dose? _____

5. Weight: 22 pounds
   Ordered dose: Ampicillin 30 milligrams per kilogram per day
   Recommended dose from drug label: 25–50 milligrams per kilogram per day in equally divided doses every 8 hours
   Does the doctor's order fit within the recommended safe guidelines?
   _____
   What is the daily dose? _____
   What is the individual dosage? _____

6. The physician orders a medication at 1.5 milligrams per kilogram over 24 hours, divided into three doses. The client weighs 78 pounds.

What is the weight in kilograms? _____
What is the daily dose? Round to the nearest whole number. _____
What is the individual dose? Round to the nearest whole number.
_____

7. The nurse is to administer the recommended dose of Garamycin 2 milligrams per kilogram every 6 hours. The child weighs 42 pounds.
   What is the weight in kilograms? _____
   What is the daily dose? Round to the nearest whole number. _____
   What is the individual dose? _____

8. The physician orders Kantrex. The recommended dose is at 2.5 milligrams per kilogram every 8 hours. The client weighs 38 pounds 4 ounces.
   What is the weight in kilograms? _____
   What is the daily dose? Round to the nearest whole number. _____
   What is the individual dose? Round to the nearest whole number.
   _____

9. The physician has ordered Proventil syrup orally at 0.1 milligrams per kilogram three times a day. The client weighs 28 pounds 8 ounces.
   What is the weight in kilograms? _____
   What is the daily dose? _____
   What is the individual dose? Round to the nearest whole tenth.
   _____

10. The physician orders a therapeutic IV medication at 2 milliliters per kilogram per dose. The client weighs 108 pounds.
    What is the weight in kilograms? _____
    What is the individual dose? _____

BASIC DOSAGE BY
BODY WEIGHT SELF-TEST

Convert the following pounds to kilograms:

Weight in pounds and ounces	Weight in kilogram
1. 14 pounds 2 ounces	_____
2. 82 pounds	_____
3. 7 pounds 15 ounces	_____
4. 8 pounds 12 ounces	_____
5. 12 pounds 10 ounces	_____
6. 33 pounds 8 ounces	_____

Calculate the dosages:
Read the following client information and medication order.

Weight: 16 pounds 6 ounces
Ordered dose: 1.2 milligrams per kilogram per day
Recommended dosage from drug label: 3 milligrams every 8 hours

7. What is the daily dose? _____

8. What is the individual dose? _____

9. Does the dose ordered match the recommended dosage? _____

Read the following client information and medication order.

Weight: 32 pounds 8 ounces
Ordered dose: 0.5 milligrams per kilogram every 4 hours prn
Recommended dosage from drug label: dosages vary, not to exceed 45 milligrams over 24 hours.

10. What is the daily dose? _____

11. What is the individual dose? _____

12. Does the ordered dose meet the recommended dosage guidelines? _____

Read the following client information and medication order.

Weight: 19 pounds
Ordered dose: 0.25 micrograms per kilogram every 8 hours
Recommended dosage from drug label: no more than 6 micrograms over 24 hours

13. What is the daily dose? _____

14. What is the individual dose? _____

15. Does the ordered dose meet the recommended dosage guidelines? _____

Math for Health Care Professionals Post-Test

Whole Number Skills

1. Find the mean of the set of numbers: 16, 4, 25, 9, 10, 9, 3, 20
   _____

2. $345 +$ _____ $+ 37 = 658$

3. $1846 - 979 =$ _____

4. $324 \times 87 =$ _____

5. $27\overline{)654} =$ _____

6. The heights of the members of Michele's family are 66 inches, 81 inches, 69 inches, 70 inches, and 64 inches. Find the range in height of the members of Michele's family. _____

7. Convert from 8:15 P.M. standard time to universal time. _____

Fraction Skills

8. Order the fractions from smallest to largest: $\frac{2}{3}, \frac{6}{7}, \frac{6}{21}, \frac{13}{21}$ _____

9. $20\frac{3}{5} + 6 + 3\frac{5}{6} =$ _____

10. $56\frac{1}{3} - 17\frac{11}{12} =$ _____

11. $2\dfrac{4}{5} \times \dfrac{2}{7} \times 5 =$ _____

12. $4\dfrac{1}{6} \div \dfrac{3}{8} =$ _____

13. Solve: $\dfrac{\dfrac{1}{10}}{\dfrac{1}{200}} =$ _____

Decimal Skills

14. Express as a fraction: 4.06 _____

15. Express as a decimal: $12\dfrac{5}{8}$ _____

16. $10.6 + 6 + 2.09 =$ _____

17. $65.7 - 12.68 =$ _____

18. $0.9 \times 41.2 =$ _____

19. $248.06 \div 0.8 =$ _____

Ratio and Proportion Skills

20. A container holds 34 milliliters of medication. How many *full* 1.25 milliliter doses can be administered from this container? _____

21. Solve: $12 : 75 :: 2.5 : x$ Round to the nearest hundredth.

    $x =$ _____

22. Solve: $8 : x :: 42 : 50$

    $x =$ _____ Answer should be in mixed number.

23. Solve: $\dfrac{1}{2} : 8 :: x : 32$ $x =$ _____

24. Solve: $\dfrac{1}{50} : 10 :: \dfrac{10}{250} : x$ $x =$ _____

25. Simplify the ratio to the lowest terms: $9\dfrac{3}{8} : 5$ _____

Percent Skills

26. What is $3\frac{2}{3}\%$ of 125? Write the answer as a mixed number. _____

27. What percent is 22 of 144? _____ Round to the nearest hundredth.

28. 24% of 250 is what number? _____

29. The original price minus a $45 discount is the sale price of a new desk. The sale price is $350. What was the original price? _____ _____

30. There are 8 grams of pure drug in 75 milliliters of solution. What is the percent strength of solution? Round to the nearest hundredth. _____

Combined Application

31. $5\frac{1}{4}$ feet = _____ inches

32. _____ quarts = $7\frac{1}{2}$ pints

33. 36 pounds = _____ kilograms

34. _____ teaspoons = 62 milliliters

35. Convert 0.7% to a fraction = _____

36. Convert $4\frac{1}{2}$ to a percent = _____

37. Convert 9 to a percent = _____

38. Write 0.002 as a fraction = _____

39. Write 0.03% as a decimal = _____

Pre-Algebra

40. $75 + (-8) =$ _____

41. $-15 - 22 =$ _____

42. $-72 \div 9 =$ _____

43. $-124 \times (-3) =$ _____

44. $21 + \sqrt{169} =$ _____

45. $(100 - 40) \div 4 =$ _____

Drug Labels

46. Complete the table for this drug label. If the information is not provided, write *Not shown*.

Fosamax® 40 mg
(Alendronate Sodium Tablets)

MERCK & CO., INC.
Whitehouse Station, NJ 08889, USA

Each tablet contains 52.21 mg Alendronate
Sodium (40 mg free acid equivalent).
Store in a well-closed container at room
temperature, 15 - 30°C (59 - 86°F).

30 Tablets

Lot

NDC 0006-0212-31

USUAL ADULT DOSAGE: 40 mg once a day
taken *at least* one-half hour before the first
food, beverage or medication of the day with
a full glass of plain water. Do not lie down
until after first food of the day.
See accompanying circular for complete
dosage information.

Rx only

9683405
30 | No. 3592

The labels for the products Prinivil, Fosamax, Singulair, Cozaar, Pepcid,
Hyzaar, and Zocor are reproduced with the permission of Merck & Co., Inc.,
copyright owner.

Generic name   _____

Trade name   _____

Manufacturer   _____

National Drug Code (NDC) number   _____

Lot number (control number)   _____

Drug form   _____

Dosage strength   _____

Usual adult dose   _____

Total amount in vial, packet, box   _____

Prescription warning   _____

Expiration date   _____

47. The medical assistant was asked to dispense 23 milliliters of a liquid
medication. Shade the medicine cup to indicate this dosage.

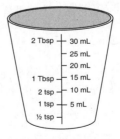

48. The physician has ordered an IM injection of 0.6 milliliters. Shade
the syringe to indicate this volume of medication.

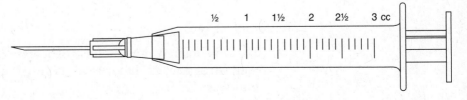

Metric Measurements

49. 9.43 micrograms = _____ milligrams

50. 193 grams = _____ kilogram. Round to the nearest tenth.

Apothecary Measurements

51. 12 fluid ounces = _____ milliliters

52. $4\frac{1}{4}$ teaspoons = _____ milliliters

53. $6\frac{1}{2}$ pints = _____ milliliters

54. 0.2 milligrams = grain _____

55. grain $\frac{1}{100}$ = _____ milligrams

56. 45 grams = grain _____

57. $4\frac{3}{4}$ teaspoons = _____ milliliters

Oral Medications

58. Desired: Aspirin 0.5 grams every 4 hours
    Available: Aspirin 500 milligrams scored tablets
    Give: _____

59. The patient is ordered Vistaril 12 milligrams orally every 6 hours for nausea relief. You have on hand Vistaril oral suspension 5 milligrams per 2.5 milliliters.
    You adminster _____.

Dosage Calculations

60. Ordered: Zocor 50 milligrams
    Have: Zocor 12.5 milligrams per tablet
    Desired dose: _____.

61. The doctor has ordered Zyloprim 0.5 gram orally twice a day. On hand is Zyloprim 100 milligrams scored tablets. The nurse should give _____.

62. The client receives an order for Augmentin 250 milligrams. The Augmentin is labeled 100 milligrams in 5 milliliters. The client will be given _____.

Parenteral Dosages

63. The physician orders megestrol acetate 600 milligrams per day. The megestrol acetate label reads, oral suspension 40 milligrams per milliliter. Give _____.

64. Give Dilaudid 0.5 milligrams IM from a vial that is labeled 5 milligrams per milliliter.
    Give _____.

65. Ordered: Atropine sulfate 0.5 milligrams IM
    Have: Atropine sulfate 0.25 milligrams per milliliter
    Give   _____

66. The doctor prescribes heparin 4000 units sub-Q four times a day. You have heparin 1500 units per milliliter. You give_____.

67. Ordered: Quinidine 0.4 gram orally every 4 hours. Quinidine is supplied in 100 milligrams tablets. How many tablets will you give?_____.

Calculating IV dosages

68. The patient with oliguria has an order for 125 milliliters of 0.9% NS over 2 hours. The drop factor is 15 drops per milliliter. How many drops per minute should be given?_____

69. The nurse receives an order that reads: 1200 milliliters D_5W IV at 60 milliliter per hour. Infuse for _____.

70. The nurse will administer an IV solution at 125 milliliter per hour for 6 hours. What is the total volume infused? _____

Basic Dosages by Body Weight

Perform the calculations to determine whether the following is a therapeutic dosage for this child:

Ordered medication XZY 5 milligrams orally every 12 hours for a child weighing 14 pounds. You have medication XYZ 10 milligrams per milliliter. The recommended daily oral dosage for a child is 1.5 milligrams per kilogram per day in divided doses every 8 hours.

```
┌─────────────────────────────────────┐
│                                       │
│            Medication XYZ             │
│            Oral Solution              │
│             10 mg/mL                  │
│                                       │
└─────────────────────────────────────┘
```

71. This child's weight is _____ kilograms.

72. What is the recommended dosage for this child?_____ milligrams per day

Weight: 24 pounds 4 ounces
Ordered dose: 1.6 milligrams per kilogram per day
Recommended dosage from drug label: 3 milligrams every 8 hours

73. What is the daily dose? _____

74. What is the individual dose? _____

75. Does the dose ordered match the recommended dosage? _____

Answers for the Post-Test

1. 12
2. 276
3. 867
4. 28,188
5. 24.22, or 24 R 6, or $24\frac{2}{9}$
6. 17
7. 0815
8. $\frac{6}{21}$, $\frac{13}{21}$, $\frac{2}{3}$, $\frac{6}{7}$
9. $30\frac{13}{30}$
10. $38\frac{5}{12}$
11. 4
12. $11\frac{1}{9}$
13. 20
14. $4\frac{3}{50}$
15. 12.625
16. 18.69
17. 53.02
18. 37.08
19. 310.075
20. 27 doses
21. 21.29
22. $9\frac{11}{24}$

23. 2
24. 20
25. 15 : 8
26. $4\frac{7}{12}$
27. 15.28
28. 60
29. $395.00
30. 10.67
31. 63
32. 15
33. 16.4
34. 14
35. 70
36. 450%
37. 900%
38. $\frac{1}{500}$
39. $\frac{3}{10,000}$
40. 67
41. −37
42. −8
43. 372
44. 34
45. 15

46.

Generic name	Alendronate sodium
Trade name	Fosamax
Manufacturer	Merck & Co., Inc.
National Drug Code (NDC) number	0006-0212-31
Lot number (control number)	Not shown
Drug form	Tablet
Dosage strength	40 milligrams
Usual adult dose	40 milligrams Once a day taken at least one-half hour before the food, beverage, or medication of the day
Total amount in vial, packet, box	30 Tablets
Prescription warning	Rx only
Expiration date	Not shown

47. 23 milliliters

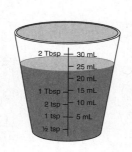

48. 0.6 milliliter

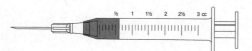

49. 0.00943 milligram

50. 0.2 kilogram

51. 360 milliliters

52. 21.25 milliliters

53. 3250 milliliters

54. grain $\frac{1}{300}$

55. 0.6 milligram

56. grain $7\frac{1}{2}$ or grain viiss

57. 23.75 milliliters

58. 1 tab

59. 6 milliliters

60. 4 tablets

61. 5 tablets

62. 12.5 milliliter

63. 15 milliliters

64. 0.1 milliliter

65. 2 milliliters

66. 2.67 milliliters

67. 4 tabs

68. 16 drops per minute

69. 20 hours

70. 750 milliliters

71. 6.36 kilograms

72. 9.54 milligrams per day

73. 18.37 milligrams per day

74. 6.12 milligrams

75. No, contact the physician for clarification.

Appendix of Practice Tests
Units 1–14

Unit 1 Practice Exam   Name _____

Solve each problem below. Place your answer on the blank line.

1. $968 + 45 + 19 =$ _____

2. $529 + 3{,}456 =$ _____

3. The heights of the people in Michele's family are 68 inches, 65 inches, 73 inches, 74 inches, and 84 inches. Find the range of the people in Michele's family. _____

4. $709 +$ _____ $+ 49 = 1670$

5. $2{,}852 - 1{,}418 =$ _____

6. $2{,}003 -$ _____ $= 907$

7. _____ $- 95 = 896$

8. $1{,}455 - 509 =$ _____

9. Write 1322 in standard time. _____

10. The dental office ordered 8 jackets for its staff. The jackets cost \$37.00 each. What is the total cost for the 8 jackets? Write a number statement to solve this problem. Include the answer. _____

11. The heights of the members of Michele's family are 69 inches, 75 inches, 70 inches, 85 inches, and 73 inches. Find the median height of the members of Michele's family. _____

12. $14 \times 3 \times 12 =$ _____

13. $45 \times 138 =$ _____

14. Divide 932 by 8 = _____

15. 5,860 ÷ 14 = _____

16. $12\overline{)907}$ = _____

17. Heather's math tests had the following scores: 98, 75, 92, 98, 76, 87, 75, and 80. What is the mode of her scores? _____

18. Each gram of fat contains 9 calories. How many grams of fat are in 144 calories of fat in a piece of steak? _____

19. Bette was working hard to get a good grade. Her test scores were: 68%, 79%, 100%, 85%, and 88%. What is the mean or average of her grades? _____

20. Round 12,885 to the nearest ten. _____

21. Use one of the symbols (=, >, <, ≤, ≥) to complete the number statement: 285 + 17 _____ 51 × 6

22. Write the Roman numeral xixss as an Arabic numeral. _____

23. After a heart attack, Bob spent two days in the coronary care unit. His bill was $4,596.00. What was his daily room rate? Write a number statement that represents this problem. _____

24. Write a number statement using the symbol (>) _____

25. Find the prime factorization for 80. _____

Unit 2 Practice Exam   Name _____

Solve each problem. Put your answer on the blank line. Correct format is necessary.

1. Make into an equivalent fraction: $\dfrac{1}{4} = \dfrac{}{36}$ _____

2. Reduce to the lowest/simplest terms: $\dfrac{3}{129} =$ _____

3. Write as an improper fraction: $12\dfrac{3}{4} =$ _____

4. Write as a mixed number: $\dfrac{235}{9} =$ _____

5. $\dfrac{4}{5} + \dfrac{3}{8} =$ _____

6. $14\dfrac{3}{4} + \dfrac{5}{6} + 2\dfrac{7}{12} =$ _____

7. $22\dfrac{1}{5} + 1\dfrac{7}{9} =$ _____

8. $48\dfrac{2}{7} - 21\dfrac{5}{21} =$ _____

9. $676 - \dfrac{3}{11} =$ _____

10. $42\dfrac{5}{12} - 17\dfrac{5}{6} =$ _____

11. $\dfrac{3}{8} \times \dfrac{5}{7} =$ _____

12. $\dfrac{7}{12} \times 8 =$ _____

13. $7\dfrac{3}{4} \times 2\dfrac{1}{3} =$ _____

14. A bottle of medicine contains 12 doses of medication. How many full doses are in $4\dfrac{1}{4}$ bottles? _____

15. $\dfrac{3}{14} \div \dfrac{1}{5} =$ _____

16. $7\dfrac{1}{8} \div 10 =$ _____

17. How many full grain $\dfrac{3}{4}$ doses can be obtained from a grain $9\dfrac{1}{2}$ vial? _____

18. $35°C =$ _____ $°F$

19. $68°F = \underline{\hspace{1cm}}°C$

20. $\dfrac{\dfrac{2}{5}}{\dfrac{1}{7}} = \underline{\hspace{1.5cm}}$

21. $\dfrac{\dfrac{1}{200}}{\dfrac{1}{6}} = \underline{\hspace{1.5cm}}$

22. Order the following the following fractions by writing them in order from smallest to largest—do not just put the number of the order on top of the fraction. $\frac{1}{2}$ $\frac{3}{4}$ $\frac{4}{9}$ $\frac{17}{36}$ $\underline{\hspace{1.5cm}}$

23. One cup holds 8 ounces. If a cup is $\frac{2}{5}$ full, how many ounces are in the cup? $\underline{\hspace{1.5cm}}$

24. The nurse gave the patient a tablet of grains $\frac{1}{20}$ of medicine followed by a second tablet of grains $\frac{5}{80}$. How many total grains of the medication did the patient receive? $\underline{\hspace{1.5cm}}$

25. The physical therapist suggested that Bob begin a series of stretches. He told Bob to work out for $\frac{1}{3}$ of an hour. How many minutes is $\frac{1}{3}$ of an hour? $\underline{\hspace{1.5cm}}$ minutes.

Unit 3 Practice Exam   Name _____

1. Write the words in decimal numbers: seven-hundredths. _____

2. Write the decimal number of 17.005 in words. _____

3. Round 25.075 to the nearest hundredth: _____

4. Which is larger: 10.07 or 10.7 = _____

5. $0.4 + 12 + 0.11 =$ _____

6. $36.05 + 1.7 + 0.009 =$ _____

7. One medication is labeled 48.5 milliliters and another is 0.5 milliliters. What is the total dosage in milliliters given of this medication? _____

8. $8.008 - 0.98 =$ _____

9. $0.9 - 0.007 =$ _____

10. Patient Smith was on a diet. He weighed 122.6 kilograms. After one month he weighed 112.8 kilograms. What was his total weight loss in one month? _____

11. $0.596 \times 2.3 =$ _____

12. $405 \times 3.02 =$ _____

13. $16\overline{)42.98}$ Round to the nearest tenth = _____

14. $1.9\overline{)28.09}$ Round to the nearest hundredth = _____

15. Change 2.85 to a fraction. Reduce if necessary. _____

16. Write $\dfrac{7}{8}$ as a decimal. _____

17. $98.5°F =$ _____ °C

18. $14°C =$ _____ °F

19. $\dfrac{12.50}{0.50} \times 4.5 =$ _____

20. Something was wrong with Tu. He felt sick, and he had a fever. At 3:00 P.M. his temperature was 101.8°F. By 5:00 P.M. it was 102.3°F. How many degrees had his temperature gone up by? _____

21. Valley Vista used a 45.6 ounce can of kidney beans in a chili casserole recipe. If each portion gets an equal amount of the beans and the recipe serves 9 people, how many ounces will each serving contain? Round to the nearest whole number. _____

22. I had an interview at the dental clinic for a dental assistant post. I had to stop to get gas. I put 7 gallons of gas in my car. Each gallon cost me $2.86. How much did I spend on gas? _____

23. The farm raises its own produce and meat. Will has a cow that produces milk. She gives 2.3 gallons of milk a day. How many gallons does she give in a month that has 30 days? _____

24. Bradley Benjamin heard that the nursing staff at Sky View earns $13.93 per hour. He is currently earning $12.46 per hour. How much more could he earn a week at Sky View than his current job if he calculated the rate for a 40 hour week? _____

25. Sally is trying to increase her dietary fiber intake. She eats 20.8 grams of fiber a day. If her goal is to eat 32 grams of dietary fiber, how many more grams of fiber does she need to eat? _____

Unit 4 Practice Exam   Name _____

Solve the ratio and proportion problems. Remember that ratios are reduced to their simplest form.

1. Write 8 days out of 15 as a ratio: _____

2. Is this an example of a proportion? Check the answer box.

    $2 : 3 :: 20 : 15$ ☐ Yes ☐ No

3. $5 : 30 = 12 : ?$ $? = $ _____

4. $\frac{1}{4} : 5 = ? : 70$ $? = $ _____

5. $82 : ? = \frac{1}{2} : 18$ $? = $ _____

6. $\frac{2}{4} = \frac{?}{98}$ $? = $ _____

7. $\dfrac{\frac{1}{2}}{\frac{1}{4}} = \dfrac{90}{?}$ $? = $ _____

8. $\frac{1}{12} : 28 = ? : 84$ $? = $ _____

9. If eggs cost \$2.10 a dozen, how much do 16 eggs cost? _____

10. If Jerry makes \$13.10 an hour, what is her pay for 15 hours? _____

11. A mouthwash cost \$4.36 for 32 ounces. How much is paid per ounce? _____

12. Each calendar for the nursing home fund raiser costs \$8.75. What is the cost for 25 calendars? _____

13. Simplify the following ratio $12\frac{1}{4} : 8$ _____

14. Simplify the following ratio $15 : \frac{1}{3}$ _____

15. Solve $^{1.7}/_{x} = {}^{8.2}/_{0.8}$ Round to the nearest tenth. _____

16. A set of three surgical masks cost \$1.39. How many complete sets of masks can you buy with a budget of ten dollars. Do not worry about tax or shipping _____

17. 17 teaspoons = _____ tablespoons

18. 1 inch = 2.5 centimeters so 17.8 inches = _____ centimeters. Round to the nearest tenth.

19. 1 kilogram = 2.2 pounds so 49 kilograms = _____ pounds

20. $\dfrac{5}{7\frac{2}{4}} = \dfrac{?}{12\frac{1}{2}}$? = _____

Thresa's Roasted Red Tomato Soup

Nutrition facts	Amount/serving	%DV*	Amount/serving	%DV*
Serving size ½ cup (120 milliliters) Condensed soup Servings about 2.5 Calories 90 Fat calories 0	Total fat 0 gram	0%	Total carbohydrates 20 grams	7%
	Saturated fat 0 gram	0%	Fiber 1 gram	4%
	Cholestrol 0 milligram	0%	Sugars 15 grams	
	Sodium 610 milligrams	30%	Protein 2 grams	
	Vitamin A 10% · Vitamin C 10% · Calcium 0% · Iron %			

*Percent daily values (%DV) are based on a 2,000 calories diet.

21. If $\frac{1}{2}$ cup of soup equals 120 milliliters, then how many milliliters are in $3\frac{1}{4}$ cups of soup? _____

22. If a can has 2.5 servings, how many cans are needed to serve 12 people? _____

23. One serving contains 90 calories, how many calories are in $4\frac{1}{2}$ servings? _____

24. 1 gram of fiber constitutes 4% of a daily dietary value. How many grams of fiber would be present in 25% of the daily value? _____

25. How many grams of carbohydrates are present if the portion meets 30% of the daily value of carbohydrates? Round to the nearest tenth if necessary. _____

Unit 5 Practice Exam   Name _____

1. Convert $3\frac{1}{4}$ to a percent. _____

2. Convert 0.625 to a percent _____

3. Convert 453 to a percent _____

4. Convert $\frac{2}{5}$ to a percent _____

5. Convert $4\frac{1}{5}$ to a percent _____

6. Convert $\frac{\frac{2}{5}}{75}$ to a percent _____

7. Convert 45% to a decimal _____

8. Convert $5\frac{1}{4}$% to a decimal _____

9. Convert $\frac{3}{4}$% to a fraction _____

10. What is 12% of 233? _____

11. Find 56% of 250 _____

12. What is $22\frac{1}{2}$% of 400? _____

13. What percent of 80 is 14? _____

14. Find 32% of 360. _____

15. What is $12\frac{2}{3}$% of 120? _____

16. $15\frac{1}{4}$% of what number is 45.75? _____

17. What is 0.9% of 34? _____

18. Write the ratio of pure drug to solution: 16% _____

19. Write the ratio of pure drug to solution: 1.08% _____

20. Write the ratio of pure drug to solution: $2\frac{2}{5}$% _____

21. There are 3 grams of pure drug are in 45 milliliters of solution. What is the percent strength of solution? _____

22. There are 35 milliliters of pure drug in 100 milliliters of solution. How many milliliters of pure drug are needed to make 85 milliliters of this solution. _____

23. Take a 8% discount from a final sales price of $120.00. The final sales price would now be _____.

24. Write as a simplified ratio of the pure drug form: $6\frac{1}{4}$% solution _____

25. Write as a simplified ratio of the pure drug form: 9% solution_____

Unit 6 Practice Exam   Name _____

1–15. Complete the table below:

Fraction	Decimal	Ratio	Percent
$\dfrac{1}{100}$	_____	_____	_____
_____	0.08	_____	_____
_____	_____	2 : 5	_____
_____	_____	_____	$5\dfrac{1}{4}\%$
_____	0.1	_____	_____

16. If 1 tablespoon is equivalent to 3 teaspoons, how many tablespoons are in 13 teaspoons? _____

17. One inch equals approximately 2.54 centimeters. If an infant is measured at 48 centimeters, how long is the infant in inches? Round to the nearest tenth. _____

18. One cup has 8 ounces. So $14\dfrac{1}{4}$ cups equals _____ ounces.

19. One teaspoon contains 5 milliliters. Nine and one-half teaspoons contains _____ milliliters.

20. If one pound contains 16 ounces, how many ounces are in 24 pounds? _____

21. If 1 kilogram equals 2.2 pounds, how many kilograms are in 70 pounds? _____

22. $3\dfrac{1}{4}$ feet = _____ inches

23. _____ quarts = 12 pints

24. 15 pounds = _____ kilograms

25. _____ teaspoons = 30 milliliters

Unit 7 Practice Exam   Name _____

Write integers for the following situations:

1. 30 degrees below 0 _____

2. A gain of 6 yards _____

Put the following sets of integers in order from least to greatest:

3. $9, -68, 53, -19$ _____ _____ _____ _____

4. $0, -34, 12, 50$ _____ _____ _____ _____

Find the absolute value:

5. $|26| =$ _____

6. $|-132| =$ _____

Solve:

7. $5 + (-10) =$ _____

8. $-8 - 52 =$ _____

9. $-36 \div 9 =$ _____

10. $-25 \times (-4) =$ _____

11. $6 \div (-3) =$ _____

12. $-3 + 28 =$ _____

13. $-19 \times (-1) =$ _____

14. $6 + (-9) =$ _____

15. $5 - (-2) =$ _____

16. $|-5 - 4| =$ _____

17. $|-2| \times 2 =$ _____

18. $18^2 =$ _____

19. $1^0 + (6)^2 =$ _____

20. $75 + (15)^2 =$ _____

21. $3^2 + 21^0 + 7^2 =$ _____

22. $2 + \sqrt{169} =$ _____

23. $\sqrt{25} + \sqrt{9} =$ _____

24. $(\sqrt{144} - \sqrt{64})^2 =$ _____

25. $(9^2 - 4^2) \div 5 =$ _____

Unit 8 Practice Test   Name _____

1. The numerical value for centi- is _____.

2. The numerical value for micro- is _____.

3. The numerical value for milli- is _____.

4. Gram and milligram are metric measures for measuring _____.

5. Liter and milliliter are metric measures for measuring _____.

Circle the correct metric notation for each:

6. Twelve and one-half kilograms

   a. $12\frac{1}{2}$ kg   b. 12.5 KG   c. 12.5 kg   d. $12\frac{1}{2}$ KG

7. One hundred five micrograms

   a. 105 mg   b. 0.105 mcg   c. 105 mcg   d. 100.5 mcg

8. Write the correct metric notation for six hundredth of a milliliter. _____

9. Write the correct metric notation for two tenths of a milligram. _____

10. Write the correct metric notation for ninety-three milligram. _____ _____

11. Write the correct metric notation for twelve hundredths of a kilogram. _____

12. 2.76 milligrams = _____ micrograms

13. 25 centimeters = _____ millimeters

14. 120.8 grams = _____ kilogram

15. _____ milligram = 4.7 micrograms

16. _____ liter = 95 milliliters

17. 12 grams = _____ milligrams

18. 9.05 milliliters = _____ liter

19. _____ gram = 10000 micrograms

20. _____ centimeters = 54 millimeters

21. 0.5 gram = _____ micrograms

22. 1200 milliliters = _____ liters

23. _____ kilogram = 23.8 grams

24. 33.7 meters = _____ millimeters

25. A newborn weighs 3090 grams. How many kilograms does it weigh? _____

Unit 9 Practice Test   Name _____

1. Look at the IV bag.

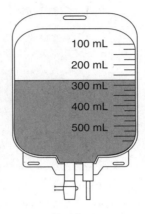

   How many milliliters have been infused?

2. Look at the label and provide the following information. If the information is not provided, write *Not shown*.

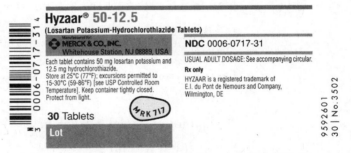

   The labels for the products Prinivil, Fosamax, Singulair, Cozaar, Pepcid, Hyzaar, and Zocor are reproduced with the permission of Merck & Co., Inc., copyright owner.

   Generic name   _____

   Trade name   _____

   Manufacturer   _____

   National Drug Code (NDC) number   _____

   Lot number (control number)   _____

   Drug form   _____

   Dosage strength   _____

   Usual adult dose   _____

   Total amount in vial, packet, box   _____

   Prescription warning   _____

   Expiration date   _____

3. Look at the label and provide the following information. If the information is not provided, write *Not shown*.

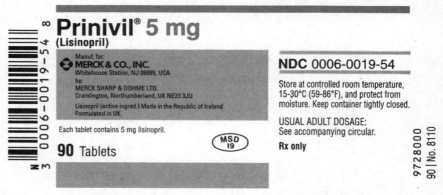

Prinivil® 5 mg
(Lisinopril)

Manuf. for:
MERCK & CO., INC.
Whitehouse Station, NJ 08889, USA
by:
MERCK SHARP & DOHME LTD.
Cramlington, Northumberland, UK NE23 3JU

Lisinopril (active ingred.) Made in the Republic of Ireland
Formulated in UK

Each tablet contains 5 mg lisinopril.

90 Tablets

MSD 19

NDC 0006-0019-54

Store at controlled room temperature,
15-30°C (59-86°F), and protect from
moisture. Keep container tightly closed.

USUAL ADULT DOSAGE:
See accompanying circular.

Rx only

9728000
90 | No. 8110

The labels for the products Prinivil, Fosamax, Singulair, Cozaar, Pepcid, Hyzaar, and Zocor are reproduced with the permission of Merck & Co., Inc., copyright owner.

Generic name   _____

Trade name   _____

Manufacturer   _____

National Drug Code (NDC) number   _____

Lot number (control number)   _____

Drug form   _____

Dosage strength   _____

Usual adult dose   _____

Total amount in vial, packet, box   _____

Prescription warning   _____

Expiration date   _____

4. The medical assistant was asked to dispense 22 milliliters of a liquid medication. Shade the medicine cup to indicate this dosage.

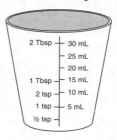

5. The physician has ordered an IM injection of 1.6 milliliters. Shade the syringe to indicate this volume of medication.

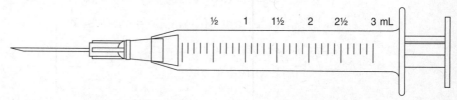

Unit 10 Practice Exam   Name _____

Make the following conversions:

1. 8 teaspoons = _____ milliliters

2. $12\frac{1}{2}$ quarts = _____ milliliters

3. grains 50 = _____ milligrams

4. 8 tablespoons = _____ milliliters

5. grain $\frac{1}{20}$ = _____ milligrams

6. 270 milligrams = grains _____

7. fluidounces 9 = _____ milliliters

8. $4\frac{1}{2}$ cups = _____ ounces

9. 200 milligrams = grains _____

10. 112 cubic centimeters = fluidounces _____

11. 0.4 milligrams = grains _____

12. $\frac{3}{4}$ cup _____ milliliters

13. 2.4 liters = _____ pints

14. 48 mg = grain _____

15. 0.3 mg = grain _____

16. A client weighs 245 pounds. What is his weight in kilograms? _____

17. The doctor orders grain iv $\frac{1}{6}$ of medication. What is the milligram equivalent of the medication order? _____

18. The dental patient is prescribed a medicated mouth rinse. He is told to swish his mouth with $2\frac{1}{2}$ tablespoons of the mouth rinse. How many milliliters of medicated mouth rinse should the patient be given? _____

19. How many tablespoons are in fluid ounces 7 of medication? _____

20. A drug packet insert states that no more than 45 milligrams of the medication should be given in a 24 hour period. How many grains is equivalent to 45 milligrams? _____

21. The client is asked to drink at least 2400 milliliters of fluid daily. How many fluid ounces is equivalent to 2400 milliliters? _____

22. The newborn baby is drinking $1\frac{3}{4}$ ounces of milk a feeding. How many tablespoons is equivalent to $1\frac{3}{4}$ ounces? _____

23. Six and one-half ounce is _____ milliliters

24. Three grams of medication is equivalent to gr. _____

25. The patient drinks $3\frac{1}{3}$ cups of tea each day. How many milliliters is $3\frac{1}{3}$ cups? _____

Unit 11 Practice Exam   Name _____

Complete the dosage calculations below using the standard conversion to find the desired dosage.

1. Ordered: Plendil 7.5 milligrams
    Have: Plendil 2.5 milligrams extended release tablets
    Desired Dose: _____

2. Ordered: Prilosec 20 milligrams
    Have: Prilosec 40 milligrams scored tablets
    Desired Dose: _____

3. Ordered: Crestor 2.5 milligrams
    Have: Crestor 5 milligrams scored tablets
    Desired Dose: _____

4. Ordered: Dilantin 100 milligrams
    Have: Dilantin 50 milligrams per tablet
    Desired Dose: _____

5. Ordered: Neurontin 500 milligrams
    Have: Neurontin 250 milligrams in 5 milliliters
    Desired Dose: _____

6. Ordered: Zocor 40 milligrams
    Have: Zocar 20 milligrams per tablet
    Desired Dose: _____

7. The doctor has ordered Zyloprim 0.25 gram orally twice a day. On hand is Zyloprim 100 milligrams scored tablets. The nurse should give _____.

8. The client receives an order for Augmentin 250 milligrams. The Augmentin is labeled 125 milligrams 5 milliliters. The client will be given _____.

9. The long-term care resident receives a medication order for albuterol sulfate liquid 4 milligrams orally three times a day. The nurse reads the albuterol sulfate liquid label and learns that each teaspoon contains 2 milligrams of the albuteral sulfate. The nurse will administer_____ teaspoons.

10. The client has a drug order for Procardia 20 milligrams three times a day. The Procardia label reads Procardia 10 milligrams per tablet. The client will receive _____ tablets three times a day.

11. Doctor Smith orders Fosamax 40 milligrams once a day taken at least 30 minutes before the first meal of the day. Read the drug label.

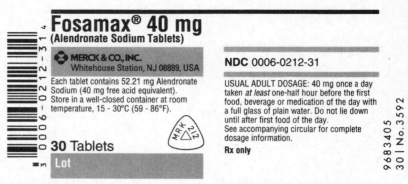

Fosamax® 40 mg
(Alendronate Sodium Tablets)

MERCK & CO., INC.
Whitehouse Station, NJ 08889, USA

Each tablet contains 52.21 mg Alendronate Sodium (40 mg free acid equivalent). Store in a well-closed container at room temperature, 15 - 30°C (59 - 86°F).

30 Tablets

Lot

NDC 0006-0212-31

USUAL ADULT DOSAGE: 40 mg once a day taken *at least* one-half hour before the first food, beverage or medication of the day with a full glass of plain water. Do not lie down until after first food of the day. See accompanying circular for complete dosage information.

Rx only

The labels for the products Prinivil, Fosamax, Singulair, Cozaar, Pepcid, Hyzaar, and Zocor are reproduced with the permission of Merck & Co., Inc., copyright owner.

The client will take _____ each day.

12. The doctor orders Cozaar 75 milligrams twice a day. The Cozaar label reads 25 milligrams per tablet. The nurse will administer _____.

13. The doctor orders Allopurinol 0.3 gram tablets orally. Allopurinol is available in 150 milligrams per tablet. Give _____.

14. Give Benedryl 75 milligrams. The vial is labeled 3 milliliters = 25 milligrams. Give _____.

15. The physician orders 200 milligrams tablets of Tagamet. On hand is 0.1 gram tabs. Give _____.

16. Give Edecrin 45 milligrams. Supply on hand is Edecrin grain $\frac{1}{4}$ tablets. Give _____.

17. The doctor orders Lanoxin 0.6 milligrams IV daily. Lanoxin is supplied in 0.4 milligrams in 2 milliliters. Give _____.

18. The patient is ordered Demerol syrup 75 milligrams orally every 4 hours as need for pain. The Demerol label reads: Demerol syrup 50 milligrams in 5 milliliters. Give _____.

19. The order reads Tylenol 0.5 gram orally every 4 hours as needed for pain. The Tylenol liquid supplied is Tylenol (acetaminophen) liquid 500 milligrams in 5 milliliters. Give _____.

20. The doctor prescribed Tagamet 150 milligrams orally. The medicine label reads Tagamet liquid 300 milligrams in 5 milliliters. How many teaspoons will be given? _____

21. A label reads Compazine 10 milliliters in 2 milliliters. The doctor prescribes an order that reads: Compazine 8 milliliters IM every 6 hours as needed for nausea. What is the individual dose? _____

22. The doctor orders Codeine grain $^1/_4$ orally every day. On hand are Codeine 30 milligrams per tablet. The nurse will give _____.

23. On hand are Phenobarbital 15 milligrams scored tablets. The order reads Phenobarbital grain $^1/_2$ orally twice a day. Give _____.

24. On hand: Slow K potassium chloride 8 milliequivalents per milliliter. The order is for potassium chloride 24 milliequivalents orally each day for prophylaxis of hypokalemia. Give _____.

25. Digoxin is available in 0.25 milligram scored tablets. The order is for digoxin 0.5 milligram orally twice a day. Give _____.

Unit 12 Practice Test   Name _____

1. The physician orders megestrol acetate 800 milligrams per day. The Megestrol acetate label reads: oral suspension 40 milligrams per milliliter. Give _____.

2. Give Dilaudid 0.5 milligram IM from a vial that is labeled 4 milligrams per milliliter. Give _____.

3. Ordered: Atropine sulfate 0.5 milligram IM
   Have: Atropine sulfate 0.3 milligram per milliliter
   Give: _____

4. The physician has ordered Calcitonin-Salmon 100 units IM for the client. The Calcitonin-Salmon vial reads 200 units per milliliter. Give _____.

5. The physician has ordered adrenalin 0.8 milligram sub-Q stat. The adrenalin label reads 1 : 1000 solution. Give _____.

6. Ordered: Cefotetan Sodium 200 milligrams IM every 24 hours piggy-back IV
   Have: Cefotetan Sodium 2 grams in 50 milliliters
   Give: _____

7. The physician has ordered magnesium sulfate 2 grams stat. The magnesium sulfate vial is labeled: 50% solution. Give _____.

8. Give Butorphanol 1.75 milligrams IV for the client every three to four hours. The Butorphanol drug label reads 1 milligram per milliliter. Give _____.

9. The physician orders Imitrex 8 milligrams sub-Q as needed for headache for the client. The Imitrex drug label on the vial reads 12 milligrams per milliliter. Give _____.

10. Ordered: Zemplar 3 micrograms IM
    Have: Zemplar 5 micrograms per milliliter
    Give: _____

11. The physician has ordered Levsin 0.25 milligram IM four times a day for the client. The drug label on the vial reads 0.5 milligram hyoscyamine sulfate injection USP per milliliter. Give_____.

12. Ordered: Lidocaine 250 milligrams sub-Q
    Have: Lidocaine 300 milligrams in 3 milliliters
    Give: _____

13. The physician has ordered Heparin 25,000 units IV from a vial that reads Heparin 10,000 units per milliliter.
    Give _____.

14. Ordered: Zantac 0.75 milligram IM stat
    Have: Zantac 0.5 milligram per milliliter
    Give: _____

15. The physician has ordered Naloxone hydrochloride 1.4 milligram IV from a vial labeled 0.4 milligram per milliliter. The nurse should administer _____.

16. The supply on hand of Morphine is grain $\frac{1}{4}$ per milliliter. The order is for Morphine sulfate 15 milligrams IM immediately. The client will receive an injection of _____.

17. The physician orders Valium 5 milligrams IM every 6 hours as needed to calm restlessness in a client. The on hand supply is Valium 10 milligrams in 2 milliliter. The nurse will administer _____.

18. The order is for Neostigmine methylsulfate 1 milligram IM sympto-matic control of Myasthenia Gravis. The supply is Neostigmine methyl-sulfate 1 : 2000. The nurse will prepare an injection of _____.

19. Ordered: Epotetin alfa 3800 units sub-Q three times a week
    Have: Epotetin alfa 4000 units per milliliter
    Give: _____

20. Ordered: Ceftin oral suspension 250 milligrams twice a day
    Have: Ceftin oral suspension 125 milligrams in 5 milliliters
    Give: _____

21. Ordered: E.E.S. 500 milligrams orally twice a day
    Have: E.E.S. oral suspension 200 milligrams in 5 milliliters
    Give: _____

22. A home resident is to have 15 milliliters of a medication to aid with digestion. A disposable medicine cup is not available. How can the dosage be measured accurately with the items in a residence? _____ What is the dosage? _____.

23. A patient is to receive a Depo-Provera 1000 milligrams IM. The vial reads Depo-Provera 400 milligrams per milliliter. Prepare _____.

24. The physician orders Zemplar 3 micrograms IM every day. The Zemplar label reads 5 micrograms per milliliter. Give an injection of _____.

25. The Neulasta label reads Neulasta 6 milligrams in 0.6 milliliter. The doctor's order reads: Give Neulasta 6 milligrams sub-Q immediately. The nurse will prepare _____.

Unit 13 Practice Test   Name _____

Complete the following calculation of IV flow rates. Round your answers to the nearest whole number.

	Amount of fluid in milliliters	Time in hours	IV Set Drop Factor	drops per minute
1.	200	3	10	_____
2.	750	12	15	_____
3.	1250	10	60	_____
4.	650	4	20	_____
5.	2000	24	60	_____

Solve each of the following problems.

6. The physician has ordered D_5W 1000 milliliters in 12 hours using a 20 drops per milliliter infusion rate. Infuse at _____ drops per minute.

7. The registered nurse is to infuse the 2 units of whole plasma (500 milliliters each) over 8 hours using a blood administration rate of 10 drops per milliliter. Infuse at _____ drops per minute.

8. The nurse reads the physician's order for 500 milliliters of D_5 $\frac{1}{4}$ NS over 12 hours at 15 drops per milliliter. Infuse at _____.

9. Infuse 550 milliliters D_5 $\frac{1}{2}$ NS over 4 hours. Use 60 drops per milliliter. Infuse at _____.

10. The nurse receives a physician's order for 250 milliliters plasma over 8 hours at 10 drops per milliliter. Infuse at _____.

11. Infuse 1000 milliliters D_5W IV in 18 hours. Infuse at _____ milliliters per hour.

12. Infuse 750 milliliters D_5 0.45% NaCl IV for 10 hours. Infuse at _____ milliliters per hour.

13. The physician orders 1000 milliliters $D_{10}W$ to infuse over 12 hours. Infuse at _____ milliliters per hour.

14. The physician's order is for D_5NS 1250 milliliters to infuse over 18 hours. Infuse at _____ milliliters per hour.

15. The nurse receives an order for 550 milliliters Normosol R over 6 hours. Infuse at _____ milliliters per hour.

16. Infuse 1000 milliliters of medication over 6 hours. Infuse at _____ milliliters per hour.

17. The nurse will administer an IV solution at 83 milliliters per hour for 8 hours. What is the total volume infused? _____

18. The patient will receive an IV therapy that runs at 150 milliliters per hour for 12 hours. What is the total volume infused? _____

19. The physician has ordered a therapeutic IV solution at 42 milliliters per hour for 18 hours. What is the total volume infused? _____

20. The nurse will administer $\frac{1}{2}$ NS IV at 75 milliliters per hour for 6 hours. What is the total volume infused? _____

21. Ordered D_5 RL IV at 83 milliliters per hour for 4 hours. What is the total volume infused? _____

22. The nurse receives an order that reads 1500 milliliters D_5W IV at 60 milliliters per hour. Infuse for _____.

23. A baby is to receive 240 milliliters D_5NS at 35 milliliters per hour. Infuse for _____.

24. Infuse 1000 D_5W milliliters at 83 milliliters per hour. Infuse for _____.

25. The patient is to receive LR 1000 milliliters at 123 milliliters per hour. Infuse for _____.

Unit 14 Practice Test   Name _____

Convert the following pounds to kilograms:

Weight in pounds and ounces	Weight in kilogram. Round to hundredth place.
1. 12 pounds 6 ounces	_____
2. 54 pounds	_____
3. 34 pounds 14 ounces	_____
4. 22 pounds 12 ounces	_____
5. 102 pounds 10 ounces	_____
6. 13 pounds 8 ounces	_____

Calculate the dosages:
Read the following client information and medication order:

Weight: 34 pounds 6 ounces
Dose ordered: 1.4 milligrams per kilogram per day
Recommended dosage from drug label: 3 milligrams every 8 hours

7. What is the daily dose? _____

8. What is the individual dose? _____

9. Does the dose ordered match the recommended dosage? _____

Read the following client information and medication order:

Weight: 26 pounds 8 ounces
Dose ordered: 0.5 milligram/kilogram every 6 hours, prn
Recommended dosage from drug label: dosages vary, not to exceed 45 milligrams per 24 hours.

10. What is the daily dose? _____

11. What is the individual dose? _____

12. Does the dose ordered meet the recommended dosage guidelines? _____

Read the following client information and medication order:

Weight: 22 pounds
Dose ordered: 0.25 microgram per kilogram every 8 hours
Recommended dosage from drug label: no more than 5 micrograms over 24 hours

13. What is the daily dose? _____

14. What is the individual dose? _____

15. Does the dose ordered meet the recommended dosage guidelines? _____

16. The order is for theophylline 55 milligrams four times a day via nasal gastric tube. The recommended dosage is 22 milligrams per kilogram every 6 hours. The child weighs 10 kilograms. Is the doctor's dosage within the recommended dosage guidelines? _____ Yes _____ No

Cefuroxine 375 milligram IV is ordered every 8 hours for a child whose weight is 45 pounds. The recommended dose is 50 milligrams per kilogram per day.

17. What is the daily dose? _____

18. What is the individual dose? _____

19. Does the dose ordered meet the recommended dosage guidelines? _____

An infant with a urinary tract infection has an order for ampicillin IV 125 milligrams every 6 hours. The infant weighs 10 pounds. The recommended dose is 50 milligrams per kilogram per day in every 6 hours.

20. What is the daily dose? _____

21. What is the individual dose? _____

22. Does the dose ordered meet the recommended dosage guidelines? _____

A 6 pound 8 ounce infant has an order for Vancomycin IV. The recommended dosage is 10 milligrams per kilogram every 12 hours for the first week of life.

23. What is the weight in kilograms?

24. What is the daily dose? _____

25. What is the individual dose? _____

Complete Answer Key for Student Work Text

Unit 1: Whole Number Review

Symbols and Number Statements
Practice 1: p. 12

1. <
3. >
5. ≥
7. >
9. >
11. ≤

Practice 2: p. 12

Answers will vary

Addition Practice: p. 13

1. 19
3. 492
5. 2,063
7. 488
9. 2,664

Addition Applications: pp. 13–14

1. a. 266
   b. 711
   c. 1,176
   d. 20 boxes
3. a. 300
   b. 720
   c. 75

d. 110
e. 1,205

Subtraction Practice: p. 15

1. 394
3. 235
5. 437
7. 1,873
9. 4,212

Subtraction Applications: p. 15

1. 1,474
3. 3 boxes

Multiplication Practice: p. 17

1. 96
3. 23,508
5. 99,960
7. 12,288
9. 92,656
11. 4,152

Multiplication Applications: p. 17

1. $3,444.00
3. $525.00

Prime Factorization: p. 18

1. $2^2 \cdot 31$
3. $2^2 \cdot 23$

Division Setup Practice: p. 19

1. $76\overline{)145}$
3. $17\overline{)49}$
5. $8\overline{)2044}$

Division Practice: p. 20

1. 94
3. 3,086 R 1
5. 311
7. 1,576 R 8
9. 23,441
11. 12,506 R 1

Division Applications: pp. 20–21

1. 13 days
3. $21
5. $1,656.00
7. 9 grams

Solving for the Unknown Number with Basic Mathematics: p. 21

Practice 1: p .21

1. 74
3. 53
5. 13

Practice 2: p. 22

1. 86
3. 560
5. 35

Practice 3: p. 22

1. 39
3. 4
5. 75

Practice 4: p. 22

1. 132
3. 3
5. 18

Rounding Practice: p. 23

1. a. 3,920
   b. 140
   c. 6,950
   d. 1,930
   e. 15,930
   f. 100
3. a. 3,000
   b. 88,000
   c. 7,000
   d. 13,000
   e. 433,000
   f. 3,000

Estimation Practice: p. 24

1. a. $194
   b. $162
   c. $112
   d. $2,914

Basics of Statistical Analysis: p. 24

Mean/Average: p. 25

1. $9
3. 5
5. 7

Median: p. 26

1. 99
3. 26
5. 9

Mode: pp. 27–28

1. 8
3. #24
5. 6 & 7

Range: pp. 28–29

1. 82
3. 360
5. 87

Roman Numerals: Concept 1
Practice: p. 30

1. 13
3. 31
5. 1001
7. xxxi
9. iss

Concept 2 Practice: p. 30

1. $9\frac{1}{2}$
3. 400
5. 99
7. xxxix
9. CCXL

Concept 3 Practice: p. 31

1. 114
3. 514
5. 89
7. 404
9. $592\frac{1}{2}$

Practice: p. 31

1. xivss
3. CXLVI
5. IM
7. CDL
9. xvii

Mixed Practice: pp. 31–32

1. 750
3. 18
5. xix
7. DCVII
9. LXVI
11. 908
13. CCCLXII
15. IM

17. 78
19. MMDXV

Time in Allied Health: p. 32
Practice Convert to Universal Time: p. 33

1. 0005
3. 0739
5. 1245
7. 1757
9. 2125

Practice in Standard Time: p. 33

1. 12:56 P.M.
3. 12:09 A.M.
5. 12:48 A.M.
7. 3:24 P.M.
9. 9:12 P.M.

Whole Number Self-Test: pp. 33–35

1. 1,075
2. 263 dollars or $263.00
3. 7 dollars
4. 66
5. 16
6. 50
7. 17
8. a. $1,500
   b. $200
   c. $150
   d. $100
   e. $375
   f. $2,325.00
9. $966.00
10. 5,780
11. 110
12. $504
13. ten thousands
14. >
15. $19\frac{1}{2}$

Unit 2: Fractions

Part to Whole Relationships: p.37

1. Three parts to four total parts
3. Seven parts to eight total parts

Equivalent Fractions Practice: p. 38

1. 6
3. 8
5. 15
7. 36
9. 54

Reducing Fractions Practice: pp. 39–40

1. $\frac{1}{7}$
3. $\frac{1}{2}$
5. $\frac{1}{4}$
7. $\frac{1}{2}$
9. $\frac{1}{3}$

Reducing Mixed Numbers Practice: p. 40

1. $13\frac{1}{4}$
3. $1\frac{1}{2}$
5. $3\frac{1}{4}$
7. $2\frac{1}{9}$
9. $6\frac{1}{2}$

Fractional Parts from Words Practice: p. 41

1. $\frac{2}{5}$

3. $\frac{1}{3}$
5. $\frac{1}{8}$

Improper Fractions to Mixed Numbers Practice: pp. 41–42

1. $7\frac{1}{2}$
3. $19\frac{1}{2}$
5. $9\frac{3}{7}$
7. $2\frac{3}{8}$
9. 1

Adding Like Denominators Practice: pp. 43–44

1. 1
3. 2
5. $\frac{7}{12}$
7. $\frac{7}{13}$
9. $22\frac{5}{6}$
11. $\frac{4}{5}$
13. 1
15. $140\frac{1}{4}$

Finding Common Denominator Practice: pp. 44–45

1. 20
3. 44
5. 25
7. 200
9. 27

Adding Unlike Fractions Practice: pp. 45–46

1. $\dfrac{17}{20}$

3. $1\dfrac{1}{9}$

5. $\dfrac{1}{2}$

7. $\dfrac{13}{21}$

9. $1\dfrac{1}{15}$

11. $1\dfrac{2}{5}$

13. $106\dfrac{8}{9}$

15. $8\dfrac{7}{8}$

Finding the Common Denominator Practice: pp. 46–47

1. 20

3. 192

5. 45

7. 36

9. 30

Adding Fractions Practice: pp. 47–48

1. $9\dfrac{11}{12}$

3. $13\dfrac{1}{2}$

5. $6\dfrac{5}{7}$

7. $18\dfrac{29}{30}$

9. $18\dfrac{9}{10}$

11. $16\dfrac{17}{27}$

13. $39\dfrac{5}{12}$

15. $13\dfrac{7}{15}$

17. $4\dfrac{7}{16}$

19. $5\dfrac{1}{2}$

Addition Applications: p. 48

1. $121\dfrac{3}{4}$

3. $1\dfrac{3}{16}$

5. $3\dfrac{5}{6}$

Ordering Fractions Practice: p. 49

1. $\dfrac{4}{12}, \dfrac{1}{4}, \dfrac{2}{9}$

3. $\dfrac{20}{50}, \dfrac{33}{100}, \dfrac{6}{25}$

Subtracting Like Fractions Practice: p. 50

1. $\dfrac{1}{9}$

3. $\dfrac{2}{11}$

5. $2\dfrac{1}{6}$

7. $45\dfrac{1}{8}$

9. $\dfrac{1}{2}$

11. $\dfrac{1}{4}$

13. $12\dfrac{1}{5}$

15. $31\dfrac{1}{9}$

17. $124\frac{1}{12}$

19. $12\frac{5}{33}$

Subtracting Mixed Numbers from Whole Numbers Practice: p. 52

1. $10\frac{1}{6}$

3. $9\frac{3}{4}$

5. $14\frac{6}{13}$

7. $5\frac{6}{7}$

9. $10\frac{2}{5}$

Subtracting Fractions Practice: pp. 52–53

1. $7\frac{13}{20}$

3. $19\frac{17}{30}$

5. $5\frac{17}{22}$

7. $111\frac{23}{30}$

9. $31\frac{5}{8}$

11. $16\frac{5}{6}$

13. $76\frac{25}{36}$

15. $6\frac{1}{2}$

Additional Practice in Subtraction with Borrowing: pp. 53–54

1. $8\frac{5}{8}$

3. $9\frac{3}{4}$

5. $11\frac{3}{4}$

7. $72\frac{5}{7}$

9. $83\frac{7}{12}$

Subtraction Application: p. 54

1. $11\frac{1}{2}$

3. $99\frac{1}{4}$

5. $3\frac{1}{2}$

Multiplication Practice: p. 55

1. $\frac{1}{16}$

3. $\frac{28}{45}$

5. $\frac{3}{35}$

7. $\frac{4}{9}$

9. $\frac{13}{66}$

Multiplication: Fractions and Whole Numbers Practice: p. 56

1. $1\frac{1}{2}$

3. $16\frac{1}{3}$

5. $5\frac{3}{5}$

7. $11\frac{2}{3}$

9. 4

Multiplication Practice: p. 58

1. $1\frac{5}{7}$

3. $\dfrac{1}{4}$

5. $\dfrac{1}{20}$

7. $\dfrac{1}{4}$

9. $\dfrac{11}{96}$

11. $\dfrac{1}{24}$

Making Improper Fractions Practice: p. 59

1. $\dfrac{33}{4}$

3. $\dfrac{88}{5}$

5. $\dfrac{27}{12}$

7. $\dfrac{32}{9}$

9. $\dfrac{53}{12}$

Multiplying Fractions: p. 61

1. $\dfrac{29}{84}$

3. $\dfrac{21}{40}$

5. $\dfrac{20}{27}$

7. $40\dfrac{1}{4}$

9. $3\dfrac{17}{20}$

Multiplication Application: pp. 61–62

1. 70 doses

3. 875 milligrams

5. $18\dfrac{3}{4}$ cups

Dividing Fractions Practice: pp. 63–64

1. $\dfrac{5}{7}$

3. $\dfrac{7}{24}$

5. 8

7. $\dfrac{1}{45}$

9. $\dfrac{1}{120}$

11. $3\dfrac{8}{9}$

13. $2\dfrac{7}{9}$

15. $4\dfrac{8}{9}$

17. $\dfrac{31}{130}$

19. $1\dfrac{47}{105}$

Division Applications: p. 64

1. $9\dfrac{3}{20}$

3. $13.30

5. 10

Celsius to Fahrenheit Temperature Conversions Practice: p. 65

1. 68

3. 77

5. 104

7. 176

Fahrenheit to Celsius Temperature Conversions Practice: p. 66

1. 40

3. 10

5. 15

7. 30

Complex Fractions Practice: p. 67

1. $\dfrac{3}{32}$

3. $\dfrac{1}{15,000}$

5. $1\dfrac{1}{5}$

7. $\dfrac{4}{5}$

9. $\dfrac{15}{16}$

Mixed Complex Fraction Problems Practice: p. 68

1. 5
3. 12
5. 1

Fraction Self-Test: pp. 68–69

1. $\dfrac{1}{4}$
2. Answers will vary: $\dfrac{2}{12}, \dfrac{3}{18}, \dfrac{4}{24}$, etc.
3. $11\dfrac{1}{11}$
4. $11\dfrac{11}{12}$
5. $39\dfrac{4}{5}$
6. $30\dfrac{13}{16}$
7. $\dfrac{4}{9}$
8. 25
9. $\dfrac{2}{12}, \dfrac{1}{4}, \dfrac{1}{3}, \dfrac{3}{8}$
10. 50
11. more
12. $\dfrac{1}{3}$
13. $\dfrac{5}{8}$
14. $\dfrac{3}{8}$
15. $26\dfrac{5}{24}$

Unit 3: Decimals

Decimals in Words: pp. 71–72

1. Seven tenths
3. Five hundredths
5. One hundred fifty and seventy-five thousands
7. One hundred nine and twenty-three thousands
9. Eighteen and eight hundredths

Words to Decimals: p. 72

1. 0.2
3. 300.002
5. 6.03

Rounding to the Nearest Tenth Practice: p. 73

1. 6.7
3. 0.8
5. 25.0 or 25
7. 0.1
9. 9.9

Rounding to the Nearest Hundredth Practice: p. 73

1. 17.33
3. 4.82
5. 0.01
7. 32.65
9. 46.09

Smaller Decimals Practice: p. 74

1. 0.89
3. 2.012
5. 0.0033

Larger Decimals Practice: p. 74

1. 0.0785
3. 0.5
5. 0.675

Ordering from Largest to Smallest Practice: pp. 74–75

1. 7.5, 7.075, 0.75, 0.7, 0.07
3. 5.55, 5.15, 5.05, 0.5, 0.05

Adding Decimals Practice: pp. 75–76

1. 38.15
3. 86.235
5. 89.2496
7. 127.52
9. 214.281

Addition Applications: p. 76

1. 4.5 milligrams
3. 226 milligrams
5. 124.54 centimeters

Subtracting Decimals Practice: p. 77

1. 0.72
3. 14.065
5. 3.5013
7. 0.175
9. 87.436

Subtraction Applications: pp. 77–78

1. 0.65 liters
3. 1.5 milligrams
5. 1.8°F

Multiplying Decimals Practice: p. 79

1. 12.6
3. 33.6
5. 128.38
7. 0.8088
9. 0.4726
11. 0.0024
13. 151.11
15. 1.65036
17. 7.632
19. 6,942.53

21. 1,342.11
23. 10.04565

Multiplication Applications: p. 80

1. $420.80
3. $1,618.20
5. $128.00

Dividing Decimals Practice: p. 81

1. 0.63
3. 0.232
5. 0.12
7. 52.4
9. 3.02

Dividing with Zeros as Placeholders Practice: p. 82

1. 1,060
3. 2.08
5. 1.099
7. 30.66
9. 0.2099

Additional Practice: p. 82

1. 5.3
3. 0.04
5. 1.39
7. 403.9

Simplified Multiplication Practice: pp. 83–84

1. 135
3. 1,257.5
5. 6
7. 12,670
9. 476
11. 13.45
13. 10.09
15. 23,850

278

Complete Answer Key for Student Work Text

Simplified Division Practice: pp. 84–85

1. 1.29
3. 12.5
5. 0.025
7. 0.158
9. 0.325
11. 10.01
13. 0.03076
15. 0.10275

Division Applications: p. 85

1. $63.25
3. 3 tablets
5. $26.24

Decimal to Fraction Conversion Practice: pp. 86–87

1. $\frac{1}{25}$
3. $6\frac{1}{4}$
5. $225\frac{1}{20}$
7. $7\frac{3}{4}$
9. $9\frac{3}{10}$

Fraction to Decimal Conversion Practice: p. 88

1. 0.5
3. 0.875
5. 0.24
7. 0.2
9. $0.83\frac{1}{3}$ or 0.083

Temperature Conversions with Decimals Practice: pp. 89–90

1. 93.2
3. 224.6
5. 107.6

7. 38
9. 53.6

Mixed Fraction and Decimal Problems Practice: p. 91

1. 2.2
3. 7.5
5. 0.168
7. 7.675

Decimal Self-Test: pp. 92–93

1. Forty-five thousandths
2. 21.75
3. 16.925
4. 4.5405
5. 90.2
6. 978.74
7. 8.018, 0.81, 0.08, 0.018
8. 1,000.9
9. 2 milligrams
10. 3 tablets
11. $\frac{1}{8}$
12. 0.26
13. 3.625
14. 39.4°C
15. 1.7

Unit 4: Ratio and Proportion

Ratios: pp. 94–95

1. 5 : 7
3. 1 : 5
5. 1 : 2

Simplifying Ratio: pp. 95–96

1. 27 : 1
3. 20 : 1
5. 2 : 1
7. 13 : 21
9. 5 : 2

Proportions: p. 96

1. No
3. Yes
5. No

Solving with Proportions Practice: p. 97

1. 7.5
3. 16
5. 27
7. 14
9. 52

Measurement Conversions Using Proportions Practice: pp. 99–100

1. $7\frac{2}{3}$
3. 8
5. 9
7. 4
9. 56
11. $2\frac{1}{2}$
13. 5
15. $1\frac{1}{2}$
17. 80
19. 5

Word Problems Using Proportions Practice: p. 101

1. 3 caplets
3. 17.5 grams
5. 28 kilograms

Solving for x in Complex Problems Practice: pp. 102–103

1. 6
3. 9.6
5. 1
7. $1\frac{1}{3}$

9. 2.4
11. 1.5

Nutrition Applications: p. 104

1. 9
3. 9
5. 48
7. 1312

pp. 104–105

1. 645
3. 220
5. 121.5

Practice with Food Labels: pp. 105–108

1. 840 milliliters
3. 405 calories
5. 42.9 grams
7. 240 calories
9. 40%
11. 11 grams
13. 1200 milliliters
15. $6\frac{1}{4}$ cups

Ratio and Proportion Self-Test: pp. 108–110

1. Answers vary.
2. 3
3. 9
4. $2\frac{2}{3}$
5. 125
6. 140 milligrams
7. 8 tablets
8. 0.3 cubic centimeters
9. $\frac{1}{75}$
10. 1.5
11. 2 minutes 10 seconds
12. 80 patients
13. 640

14. $\dfrac{4}{125}$

15. 96 ounces

Unit 5: Percents

Percent-to-Decimal Practice: p. 112

1. 0.45

3. $0.78\dfrac{1}{5}$ or 0.782

5. $0.44\dfrac{1}{2}$ or 0.445

Decimal-to-Percent Practice: pp. 112–113

1. 62.5%

3. 860%

5. 7.6%

Mixed Practice: p. 113

1. 0.7689

3. 0.86

5. 7.8%

7. $125\dfrac{1}{4}\%$ or 125.25%

9. 0.015

Set Up of Percents Practice: p. 114

1. $\dfrac{25}{100} = \dfrac{x}{200}$

3. $\dfrac{8.5}{100} = \dfrac{x}{224}$

5. $\dfrac{x}{100} = \dfrac{18}{150}$

7. $\dfrac{x}{100} = \dfrac{75}{90}$

9. $\dfrac{50}{100} = \dfrac{75}{x}$

Percents Practice: p. 115

1. 18

3. 25%

5. 5.88

7. 22.5%

9. 17.60

More Complex Percents Practice: p. 116

1. 41.67

3. 60

5. 15.63

7. 1280

9. 533.33

Percent Strength Practice: p. 117

1. 1 gram of pure drug to 25 milliliters of solution

3. 1.5 grams of pure drug to 100 milliliters of solution

5. 1 gram of pure drug to 20 milliliters of solution

Percent Equivalents in Solutions Practice: pp. 118–119

1. a. 1.25 grams
   b. 1.75 grams
   c. 3.25 grams
   d. 6.25 grams

3. a. 30%
   b. 60 grams

Additional Practice with Solution Strength: pp. 119–120

1. a. 12.75 grams
   b. 100 milliliters
   c. 51 : 400
   d. 4.5 grams
   e. 10.2 grams
   f. 7.7 grams

3. a. 78 grams
   b. 100 milliliters
   c. 39 : 50
   d. 51.1 grams
   e. 70.2 grams
   f. 351 grams

Single Trade Discounts Practice: p. 121

1. $71.33 $404.17
3. $15.69 $109.86
5. $88.23 $264.67
7. $112.68 $137.72
9. $63.20 $94.80

Percent Self-Test: pp. 121–123

1. Answers vary. A percent is a number which is part of a whole. 75% is 75 parts of 100.

2. a. $87\frac{1}{4}\%$ or 87.25%

   b. $83\frac{1}{3}\%$

3. 243.75
4. 20
5. 200
6. There are 5.5 grams of pure drug in 100 milliliters of solution.
7. 2.25 grams of pure drug
8. a. $15.54
   b. $113.96

9. 8.3% or $8\frac{1}{3}\%$

10. $48.90
11. 12%
12. 2.5
13. 6.4%
14. 0.15
15. 70000

Unit 6: Combined Applications

Conversions: pp. 127–128

Fraction	Decimal	Ratio	Percent
1. $\frac{3}{4}$	0.75	3 : 4	75%
3. $\frac{1}{2}$	0.5	1 : 2	50%
5. $\frac{1}{250}$	0.004	1 : 250	0.4%

7. $\frac{3}{50}$	0.06	3 : 50	6%
9. $\frac{1}{10}$	0.1	1 : 10	10%
11. $1\frac{9}{25}$	1.36	34 : 25	136%
13. $\frac{2}{5}$	0.4	2 : 5	40%
15. $\frac{16}{25}$	0.64	16 : 25	64%
17. $\frac{5}{6}$	$0.83\frac{1}{3}$	5 : 6	$83\frac{1}{3}\%$
19. $\frac{1}{100}$	0.01	1 : 100	1%

Using Combined Application in Measurement Convertions Abbreviations: p. 129

1. Foot
3. Ounce
5. Pound
7. Quart
9. Drop

Standard Units of Measurement Conversion Review: p. 130

1. $2\frac{1}{2}$
3. 31.25 or 31.75
5. 3
7. 24
9. $2\frac{1}{2}$

More Combined Applications Practice: p. 131

1. 6
3. 36
5. 32
7. 149.6
9. 4

Mixed Review Practice: p. 132

1. 2

3. $\frac{1}{12}$

5. $\frac{1}{30}$

Converting among Systems: pp. 132–133

	Fraction	Decimal	Ratio	Percent
1.	$\frac{7}{8}$	0.875	7 : 8	$87\frac{1}{2}\%$
3.	$\frac{3}{4}$	0.75	3 : 4	75%
5.	$\frac{2}{5}$	0.40	2 : 5	40%
7.	$\frac{2}{25}$	0.08	2 : 25	8%
9.	$\frac{3}{5}$	0.6	3 : 5	60%
11.	$1\frac{5}{8}$	1.625	13 : 8	162.5%
13.	$\frac{11}{50}$	0.22	11 : 50	22%
15.	$\frac{3}{25}$	0.12	3 : 25	12%
17.	$\frac{1}{6}$	$0.16\frac{2}{3}$	1 : 6	$16\frac{2}{3}\%$
19.	$\frac{1}{25}$	0.04	1 : 25	4%

Combined Application Self-Test: pp. 133–134

1. 0.04
2. 1 : 200
3. $1\frac{1}{20}$
4. 33 : 8
5. 27.25
6. 6%
7. 57 : 400
8. 26

9. 24
10. 105 or 106.68
11. 1,080
12. 16
13. 420
14. 0.0804
15. 0.3

Unit 7: Pre-Algebra Basics

Integers: p. 136

1. +25
3. +2000
5. −12

Opposite of Integers: p. 136

1. +34
3. −5
5. −17

Examples in Health care: p. 136

1. Answers will vary

Comparing Integers: p. 137

1. >
3. >
5. <

Absolute Value: p. 138

1. 4
3. 6
5. 476

Adding Integers with Like Signs: p. 139

1. 11
3. −8
5. −66
7. 21
9. −22

Adding Integers with Unlike Signs: p. 140

1. 5

3. 15

5. 6

7. −10

9. 84

Subtracting Integers: p. 141

1. 19

3. −4

5. 20

7. 22

9. −24

Multiplication of Integers: p. 142

1. −36

3. −128

5. −230

7. −40

9. −24

Division of Integers: p. 143

1. 12

3. −82

5. −6

7. −4.2

9. −6

Exponential Notation: p. 144

1. $8 \cdot 8 \cdot 8, 512$

3. $4^2, 4 \cdot 4$

5. $7 \cdot 7, 49$

7. $1, 1$

9. $6^0, 1$

Scientific Notation: p. 145

1. 6×10^3

3. 8×10^6

5. 7.22×10^{-2}

Standard Form: p. 146

1. 10,300

3. 90,000,000

5. 0.000066

7. 965,000

Square Roots: p. 146

1. 4

3. 9

5. 11

7. 14

9. 17

Order of Operations: pp. 147–148

1. 40

3. 11

5. 11

7. −32

9. 9

Algebraic Expressions: p. 148

1. $a^3, 2$

3. $x, 1.5$

5. $ab^2c, 12$

7. $bc^3, 2$

9. $bc, -7$

Algebraic Expression: p. 149

1. $c - 1.5$

3. $a + b$

5. $\dfrac{a + b}{6}$

7. $\dfrac{r}{3}$

9. $2(m + n)$

Algebraic Expressions in Words: p. 149

1. some number a plus some number b decreased by some number z

3. some number x divided by some number y decreased by 15

5. the product of 7, a, and b decreased by 15

Using Substitution: p. 150

1. 100

3. 26

5. 11

Evaluate each Expression: pp. 150–151

1. 29.75

3. $4\frac{1}{2}$

5. 40

7. 80

9. −1

Writing Expressions from Word Problems: p. 152

1. $x - 2$

3. $x + 500$

5. $x - 12$

Solving the Equations: p. 153

1. 57.5

3. 41.5

5. −12.25

7. −129.6

9. −16.4

Writing Equations from Word Problems: pp. 154–156

1. $123 + 1357 = x$ $x = 1480$

3. $(2 \cdot 16.5) + 2 = x$ $x = 35$

5. $x + 7 = 18$ $x = 11$

7. $4x + 7 = 31$ $x = 6$

9. $125 + 325 + x = 625.35$ $x = 175.35$

Literal Equations: p. 157

1. $t = \dfrac{i}{p}$

3. $s = \dfrac{p}{4}$

5. $w = b(h)$

Pre-Algebra Basics Self-Test: pp. 157–158

1. −1

2. −24

3. 33

4. 10

5. 17

6. 15552

7. 11

8. 60

9. 68

10. −2

11. 4

12. $\dfrac{y}{5}$

13. −97.6

14. $1,384.50

15. 21

Unit 8: The Metric System

Metric System: Units Practice: p. 161

1. kg

3. g

5. cm

7. km

9. liter

11. kilometer

13. mcg or μg

15. centimeter

Metric Conversions: p. 162

1. 0.004

3. 9250

5. 0.001

7. 0.3586

9. 0.0375

Conversion Practice: pp. 162–165

1. 1

3. 0.026

5. 19500

7. 300

9. 70

11. 0.14

13. 0.25

15. 600

17. 36000
19. 7.5
21. 12500
23. 240
25. 12760
27. 235
29. 0.8
31. 1
33. 125
35. 125
37. 45.25
39. 0.001
41. 5.524
43. 125
45. 90
47. 100
49. 8.5

Practice with Word Problems: pp. 165–166

1. 44.53 centimeters
3. 1890 liters, 10 servings

5. 1250 cubic centimeters
7. 123.56 centimeters, 1.2356 meters
9. Yes, 0.03 grams converts to 30 milligrams

Metric Self-Test: pp. 166–167

1. 250000
2. 0.075
3. 0.0546
4. 8300
5. 14000
6. 0.0012
7. 0.00001
8. 0.25
9. 15
10. 30000
11. 0.000008 milligrams
12. 34.5 centimeters
13. 7.5 milliliters
14. 240 milliliters
15. 750 milligrams

Unit 9: Reading Drug Labels, Medicine Cups, Syringes, and Intravenous Fluid Administration Bags

Practice: pp 169–173

1.
Generic name	Famotidine
Trade name	Pepcid
Manufacturer	Merck & Co., Inc.
National Drug Code (NDC) number	0006-0963-31
Lot number (control number)	Not shown
Drug form	Tablet
Dosage strength	20 milligrams
Usual adult dose	Not shown, see accompanying circular
Total amount in vial, packet, box	30 tablets
Prescription warning	Rx only
Expiration date	Not shown

3.
Generic name	Sertraline HCl
Trade name	Zoloft
Manufacturer	Pfizer Roerig

National Drug Code (NDC) number	0049-4960-30
Lot number (control number)	Not shown
Drug form	Tablet
Dosage strength	25 milligrams
Usual adult dose	Not shown, see accompanying prescribing information
Total amount in vial, packet, box	30 tablets
Prescription warning	Rx only
Expiration date	Not shown

5.

Generic name	Olanzapine
Trade name	ZyPREXA
Manufacturer	Eli Lilly and Company
National Drug Code (NDC) number	0002-4115-60
Lot number (control number)	Not shown
Drug form	Tablet
Dosage strength	5 milligrams
Usual adult dose	Not shown, see accompanying literature for dosage
Total amount in vial, packet, box	60 tablets
Prescription warning	Rx only
Expiration date	Not shown

Practice with medicine cups: p. 173

1. 2 teaspoons or 10 milliliters
3. 2 tablespoons or 30 milliliters

Practice with Syringes: pp. 173–174

1. 0.8 cubic centimeters

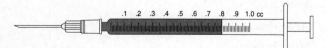

3. 0.35 cubic centimeters

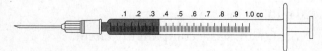

5. 5.8 milliliters

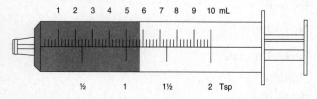

Practice with IV administration bags: p. 175

1.	Volume infused	350 milliliters
	Volume remaining	150 milliliters
3.	Volume infused	150 milliliters
	Volume remaining	100 milliliters

Reading Drug Labels, Medicine Cups, Syringes, and Intravenous Fluid Administration Bags Self-Test: pp. 175–177

1. Answers will vary. The generic indicates the drug is not protected by trademark. It is nonproprietary. The trade name is a brand name and these are the market names of the drug.

2. Generic name   Amlodipine besylate
   Trade name   Norvasc
   Manufacturer   Pfizer Labs
   National Drug Code (NDC) number   0069-1540-68
   Lot number (control number)   Not shown
   Drug form   Tablet
   Dosage strength   10 milligrams
   Usual adult dose   Not shown, see accompanying prescribing information

   Total amount in vial, packet, box   90 tablets
   Prescription warning   Rx only
   Expiration date   Not shown

3. 7.5 milliliters

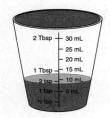

4. 1.2 milliliters

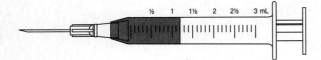

5. Volume infused   375 milliliters
   Volume remaining   625 milliliters

Unit 10: Apothecary Measurement and Conversion

Practice: p. 182

1. ss
3. $1\frac{1}{4}$
5. 10
7. 250
9. $\frac{1}{200}$
11. 210

Apothecary Equivalents Practice: p. 183

1. 900, 0.9
3. $\frac{1}{4}$, 15
5. 15, 15,000
7. 90, 0.09
9. 510, 0.51

Liquid Apothecary Equivalents Practice: pp. 183–184

1. 6
3. 15
5. 1
7. iss
9. 4
11. 2500
13. 5
15. 64
17. 75
19. 4

Mixed Apothecary Applications: pp. 184–185

1. 30
3. 62.5
5. 2250
7. 420

9. 7

11. 480

13. $\frac{1}{200}$

15. 20

17. $\frac{1}{2}$

19. 300

21. 0.4

23. ii

25. 420

27. 12

29. 35 or 35.56

31. v

33. 6

35. 4

37. 25

39. 36

Apothecary Conversions Practice: pp. 185–186

1. x

3. 4

5. 75

7. 4

9. 900

11. 8

13. 4500

15. $\frac{1}{600}$

17. $4\frac{1}{2}$

19. 312.5

21. 120

23. 24

25. 875

Rounding in Dosages: p. 187

1. 25.9 kilograms

3. 12.5 milligrams

5. 50.5 milligrams

Additional Practice with Apothecary Conversions: pp. 187–188

1. $1\frac{3}{10}$

3. $\frac{1}{2}$

5. 255

7. 0.9

9. 600

11. x or 10

13. 120

15. 75

Apothecary System Self-Test: p. 188

1. grains viiss or grains $7\frac{1}{2}$

2. v or 5

3. $\frac{1}{200}$

4. 150

5. 120

6. 105.6 or $105\frac{3}{5}$

7. $6\frac{1}{3}$

8. 0.6

9. $\frac{13}{20}$

10. 23

11. 225

12. 31.1

13. $2\frac{2}{5}$

14. 1920

15. 90

Unit 11: Dosage Calculations

Practice: pp. 193–194

1. 3 tablets

3. 3 tablets

5. 0.5 milliliter

7. 0.5 milliliter

9. 6 tablets

Two-step Dosage Calculations Practice: pp. 194–195

1. 40 milliliters

3. $\frac{1}{2}$ caplet

5. 4 tablets

7. $1\frac{1}{2}$ tablets

9. 2 tablets

More Dosage Calculation Practice: p. 195

1. $2\frac{1}{2}$ tabs

3. 2 caps

5. 2.5 tabs

7. $\frac{1}{2}$ tab

9. 4 tabs

Practice with Drug Labels: pp. 196–199

1. 1 tab

3. 2 tabs

5. 2 tabs

7. 2 tabs

9. 1 tab

Dosage Calculation Self-Test: pp. 199–201

1. 10 milliliters

2. $2\frac{1}{2}$ tabs

3. 2 tabs

4. 25 milliliters

5. 1 cap

6. 2 tabs

7. 3 tabs

8. 1 tab

9. 8 milliliters

10. 3 tabs

11. 20 milliliters

12. 2 tabs

13. 2 tabs

14. 1 milligram

15. 2 tabs

Unit 12: Parenteral Dosage

Practice: pp. 205–206

1. 0.5 milliliters

3. 2.22 milliliters = 2.2 milliliters

5. 2.5 milliliters

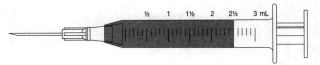

7. 2 milliliters

9. 0.5 milliliters

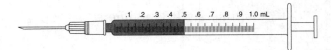

Additional Practice: p. 207

1. 0.5 milliliters

3. 0.75 milliliters = 0.8 milliliter

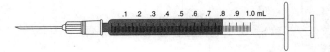

5. 2 milliliters

7. 1.5 milliliters

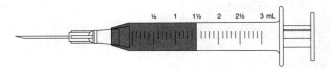

9. 0.25 milliliters = 0.3 milliliters

Parental Dosages Self-test: pp. 208–209

1. 0.6 milliliters

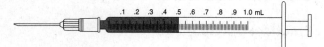

2. 0.25 milliliters = 0.3 milliliters
3. 0.75 milliliters = 0.8 milliliters

4. 0.5 milliliters

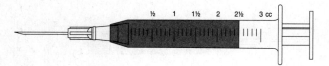

5. 0.5 milliliters
6. 2.5 cubic centimeters

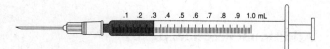

7. 2.75 milliliters = 2.8 milliliters
8. 0.33 milliliters = 0.3 milliliters
9. 0.33 milliliters = 0.3 milliliters

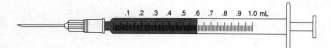

10. 0.6 milliliters

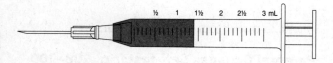

11. 2 milliliters
12. 0.5 milliliters
13. 25 milliliters
14. 1.4 milliliters

15. 0.5 milliliters

Unit 13: The Basics of Intravenous Fluid Administration

Practice: pp. 213–214

1. 100 drops per minute
3. 7 drops per minute
5. 104 drops per minute
7. 24 drops per minute
9. 17 drops per minute
11. 133 drops per minute
13. 25 drops per minute
15. 6 drops per minute
17. 84 drops per minute
19. 44 drops per minute

Additional Practice: pp. 214–215

1. 31 drops per minute
3. 21 drops per minute
5. 6 drops per minute
7. 125 drops per minute
9. 10 drops per minute

Practice: pp. 216–217

1. 83 milliliters per hour
3. 300 milliliters per hour
5. 111 milliliters per hour
7. 125 milliliters per hour
9. 75 milliliters per hour

Practice: pp. 218–219

1. 10 hours
3. 16 hours
5. 4 hours 48 minutes
7. 7 hours 50 minutes
9. 9 hours 2 minutes

Practice: p. 220

1. 1500 milliliters
3. 498 milliliters
5. 558 milliliters

7. 268 milliliters

9. 400 milliliters

The Basics of Intravenous Fluid Adminstration Self-Test: pp. 220–221

1. 16 drops per minute

2. 14 drops per minute

3. 125 drops per minute

4. 31 drops per minute

5. 94 drops per minute

6. 200 milliliters per hour

7. 63 milliliters per hour

8. 63 milliliters per hour

9. 75 milliliters per hour

10. 200 milliliters per hour

11. 4 hours

12. 4 hours 53 minutes

13. 20 hours

14. 10 hours

15. 3 hours 6 minutes

16. 810 milliliters

17. 664 milliliters

18. 75 milliliters

19. 1500 milliliters

20. 163 milliliters

Unit 14: Basic Dosage by Body Weight

Practice: p. 223

1. 6.36 kilograms

3. 12.27 kilograms

5. 18.18 kilograms

7. 7.27 kilograms

9. 13.64 kilograms

Practice: p. 224

1. 14.5, 6.59 kilograms

3. 16.25, 7.39 kilograms

5. 42.13, 19.15 kilograms

7. 12.75, 5.80 kilograms

9. 124.88, 56.76 kilograms

Practice: pp. 227–228

1. 3.92 kilograms, 58.8 milligrams

3. 8.18 kilograms, 2 milliliters

5. Yes, 300 milligrams, 100 milligrams

7. 19.09 kilograms, 152 milligrams, 38 milligrams

9. 12.95 kilograms, 3.9 milliliters, 1.3 milliliters

Basic Dosage by Weight Self-Test: pp. 228–229

1. 6.42 kilograms

2. 37.27 kilograms

3. 3.61 kilograms

4. 3.98 kilograms

5. 5.74 kilograms

6. 15.23 kilograms

7. 8.9 milligrams

8. 3 milligrams

9. Yes

10. 44.32 milligrams

11. 7.39 milligrams

12. Yes

13. 6.48 micrograms

14. 2.16 micrograms

15. No, contact the physician for clarification.

Practice Exam Answer Key

Unit 1: pp. 240–241

1. 1,032
2. 3,985
3. 16
4. 912
5. 2,346
6. 1,096
7. 991
8. 946
9. 1:22 P.M.
10. $8 \times \$37.00 = \$296.00$—May vary in format.
11. 73 inches
12. 504
13. 6,210
14. 7,456
15. 418 R 8
16. 75 R 7
17. 75 & 98
18. 16 grams
19. 84%
20. 12,890
21. $<$
22. $19\frac{1}{2}$
23. $\$4,596 \div 2 = \$2,298$
24. Answers will vary. $7 > 4$
25. $2^4 \times 5$

Unit 2: pp. 242–243

1. $\frac{9}{36}$
2. $\frac{1}{43}$
3. $\frac{51}{4}$
4. $26\frac{1}{9}$
5. $1\frac{7}{40}$
6. $18\frac{1}{6}$
7. $23\frac{44}{45}$
8. $27\frac{1}{21}$
9. $675\frac{8}{11}$
10. $24\frac{7}{12}$
11. $\frac{15}{56}$
12. $4\frac{2}{3}$
13. $18\frac{1}{12}$
14. 51 doses
15. $1\frac{1}{14}$
16. $\frac{57}{80}$
17. 12 doses
18. 95°F
19. 20°C
20. $2\frac{4}{5}$
21. $\frac{3}{100}$
22. $\frac{4}{8}, \frac{17}{36}, \frac{1}{2}, \frac{3}{4}$
23. $3\frac{1}{5}$
24. $\frac{9}{80}$
25. 20 minutes

Unit 3: pp. 244–245

1. 0.07
2. Seventeen and five thousandths
3. 25.08
4. 10.7 should be circled
5. 12.51
6. 37.759
7. 49 milliliters
8. 7.028
9. 0.893
10. 9.8
11. 1.3708
12. 1223.10
13. 2.7
14. 14.78
15. $2\frac{17}{20}$
16. 0.875
17. 36.8
18. 57.2
19. 112.5
20. 0.5°F
21. 5 ounces
22. $20.02
23. 69 gallons
24. $58.80
25. 11.2 grams

Unit 4: pp. 246–247

1. 8 : 15
2. No
3. 72
4. 3.5
5. 2952
6. 49
7. 45
8. $\frac{1}{4}$ or 0.25

9. $2.80
10. $196.50
11. $0.14 or 14¢
12. $218.75
13. 49 : 32
14. 45 : 1
15. 0.2
16. 7 sets
17. $5\frac{2}{3}$
18. 7.12
19. 107.8 or $107\frac{4}{5}$
20. $8\frac{1}{3}$
21. 780 milliliters
22. $4\frac{4}{5}$ cans
23. 405 calories
24. 6.25 grams
25. 85.7 grams

Unit 5: pp. 248–249

1. 325%
2. $62\frac{1}{2}$% or 62.5%
3. 45300%
4. 40%
5. 420%
6. 3.2%
7. 0.45
8. 0.0525
9. $\frac{3}{400}$
10. 27.96
11. 140
12. 90
13. 17.5%
14. 115.20

15. 15.20
16. 300
17. 0.306
18. 4 : 25
19. 27 : 2500
20. 3 : 125
21. $6\frac{2}{3}$% or 6.67%
22. 29.75
23. $110.40
24. 1 : 16
25. 9 : 100

Unit 6: p. 250

1–15.

Fraction	Decimal	Ratio	Percent
$\frac{1}{100}$	0.01	1 : 100	1
$\frac{2}{25}$	0.08	2 : 25	8
$\frac{2}{5}$	0.4	2 : 5	40
$\frac{21}{400}$	0.0525	21 : 400	$5\frac{1}{4}$
$\frac{1}{10}$	0.1	1 : 10	10

16. $4\frac{1}{3}$ tablespoons
17. 18.9 inches
18. 116 ounces
19. 47.5 milliliters
20. $1\frac{1}{2}$ pounds
21. 31.8 kilograms
22. 39 inches
23. 6 quarts

24. 6.8 kilograms
25. 6 teaspoons

Unit 7: pp. 251–252

1. -30
2. $+6$
3. $-68, -19, 9, 53$
4. $-34, 0, 12, 50$
5. 26
6. 132
7. -5
8. -60
9. -4
10. 100
11. -2
12. 25
13. 19
14. -3
15. 7
16. 9
17. 4
18. 324
19. 37
20. 300
21. 59
22. 15
23. 8
24. 16
25. 13

Unit 8: pp. 253–254

1. 100
2. 1000000
3. 1000
4. Weight
5. Volume
6. c. 12.5 kilograms

7. c. 105 micrograms
8. 0.06 milliliter
9. 0.2 milligram
10. 0.093 milligram
11. 0.12 kilogram
12. 0.00276
13. 250
14. 0.1208
15. 0.0047
16. 0.095

17. 12000
18. 0.00905
19. 0.01
20. 5.4
21. 500000
22. 1.2
23. 0.0238
24. 3370
25. 3.1 kilogram

Unit 9: pp. 255–256

1. 175 milliliters

2.

Generic name	Losartan Potassium-Hydrochlorthiazide
Trade name	Hyzaar
Manufacturer	Merck and Co., Inc.
National Drug Code (NDC) number	006-0717-31
Lot number (control number)	Not shown
Drug form	Tablets
Dosage strength	50–12.5 milligrams
Usual adult dose	Not shown. See accompanying circular.
Total amount in vial, packet, box	30 tablets
Prescription warning	Rx only
Expiration date	Not shown

3.

Generic name	Lisinopril
Trade name	Prinivil
Manufacturer	Merck and Co., Inc.
National Drug Code (NDC) number	006-0019-54
Lot number (control number)	Not shown
Drug form	Tablets
Dosage strength	5 milligrams
Usual adult dose	Not shown. See accompanying circular.
Total amount in vial, packet, box	90 tablets
Prescription warning	Rx only
Expiration date	Not shown

4. 22 milliliters of a liquid medication.

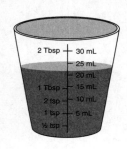

5. injection of 1.6 milliliters

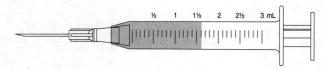

Unit 10: pp. 257–258

1. 40 milliliters
2. 12 500 milliliters
3. 3 000 milligrams
4. 120 milliliters
5. 3 milligrams
6. grains $4\frac{1}{2}$
7. 270 milliliters
8. 36 ounces
9. 3 grains $\frac{1}{3}$
10. fluidounces $3\frac{11}{15}$
11. grains $\frac{1}{150}$
12. 180 milliliters
13. $4\frac{4}{5}$ pints
14. grain $\frac{4}{5}$
15. grain $\frac{1}{200}$
16. 111.4 kilograms
17. 250 milligrams
18. 37.5 milliliters

19. fluid ounces 14
20. grain $\frac{3}{4}$
21. fluid ounces 80
22. $3\frac{1}{2}$ tablespoons
23. 195 milliliters
24. grains 50
25. 800 milliliters

Unit 11: pp. 259–261

1. 3 tablets
2. $\frac{1}{2}$ tablet
3. $\frac{1}{2}$ tablet
4. 2 tablets
5. 10 milliliters
6. 2 tablets
7. $2\frac{1}{2}$ tablets
8. 10 milliliters
9. 2 teaspoons
10. 2 tablets
11. 1 tablet
12. 3 tablets
13. 2 tablets
14. 9 milliliters
15. 2 tablets
16. 3 tablets
17. 3 milliliters
18. 7.5 milliliters
19. 5 milliliters
20. $2\frac{1}{2}$ teaspoons
21. 1.6 milliliters
22. $\frac{1}{2}$ tablet
23. $\frac{1}{2}$ tablet

24. 0.3 milliliters
25. 2 tablets

Unit 12: pp. 262–264

1. 20 milliliters
2. 0.125 milliliters
3. 1.67 milliliters
4. 0.5 milliliters
5. 0.8 milliliters
6. 0.02 milliliters
7. 4 milliliters
8. 1.75 milliliters
9. 0.67 milliliters
10. 0.6 milliliters
11. 0.5 milliliters
12. 2.5 milliliters
13. 2.5 milliliters
14. 1.5 milliliters
15. 3.5 milliliters
16. 1 milliliter
17. 1 milliliter
18. 2 milliliters
19. 0.95 milliliter
20. 10 milliliters
21. 12.5 milliliters
22. Tablespoons or teaspoons; 1 Tablespoon or 3 teaspoons
23. 2.5 milliliters
24. 0.6 milliliters
25. 0.6 milliliters

Unit 13: pp. 265–266

1. 11 drops per minute
2. 16 drops per minute
3. 125 drops per minute
4. 54 drops per minute
5. 83 drops per minute
6. 28 drops per minute
7. 21 drops per minute

8. 10 drops per minute
9. 138 drops per minute
10. 5 drops per minute
11. 56 milliliters/hour
12. 75 milliliters/hour
13. 83 milliliters/hour
14. 69 milliliters/hour
15. 92 milliliters/hour
16. 167 milliliters/hour
17. 664 milliliters
18. 1800 milliliters
19. 756 milliliters
20. 450 milliliters
21. 332 milliliters
22. 25 hours
23. 6 hours 51 minutes
24. 12 hours 3 minutes
25. 8 hours 8 minutes

Unit 14: pp. 267–268

1. 5.63 kilograms
2. 24.55 kilograms
3. 15.85 kilograms
4. 10.34 kilograms
5. 46.65 kilograms
6. 6.14 kilograms
7. 21.8 milligrams per day
8. 7.3 milligrams per dose
9. No, contact the physician for clarification.
10. 24 milligrams per day
11. 6 milligrams every 6 hours
12. Yes
13. 7.5 milligrams per day
14. 2.5 micrograms every 8 hours
15. No, contact the physician for clarification.
16. No
17. 1125 milligrams per day
18. 375 milligrams every 8 hours

19. No, too high. Contact physician for clarification.

20. 125 milligrams every 6 hours

21. 227.5 milligrams per day

22. No, recommended dose is 227.5 milligrams per day. Contact the physician for clarification.

23. 2.95 kilograms

24. 29.55 milligrams over 12 hours

25. 59.1 milligrams

Index

Rounding Guidelines

To the Tenth

Temperature in Fahrenheit and Celsius

Pounds & Kilogram

To the Hundredth

Certain medications and syringe dosages

Kilograms used for dosage by weight

Money

Common Abbreviations IV Administration

Term for IVs	Abbreviation	Term for IVs	Abbreviation
intravenous	IV	water	H_2O, W
piggy-back	PB	5% Dextrose water	D_5W
drop/drops	gtt/gtts	10% Dextrose water	$D_{10}W$
hour	hr	Normal Saline (0.9%)	NS
minutes	min	One half Normal saline (0.45%)	$\frac{1}{2}$ NS
drops per minute	gtts/min		
drops per milliliter	gtts/mL	Ringer's Lactate Solution	RL
milliliters per hour	mL/hr	Lactated Ringer's Solution	LR

Abbreviation used in Dosage

Abbreviation	Term	Abbreviation	Term
po	by mouth or orally	cap	capsule
susp	suspension	q	every
prn	as needed	bid	twice a day
tab	tablet	tid	three times a day